DATE DUE

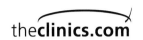

NURSING CLINICS
OF NORTH AMERICA

Advances in Endocrine Disorders

GUEST EDITOR
June Hart Romeo, PhD, NP-C

March 2007 • Volume 42 • Number 1

SAUNDERS

An Imprint of Elsevier, Inc.

PHILADELPHIA   LONDON   TORONTO   MONTREAL   SYDNEY   TOKYO

W.B. SAUNDERS COMPANY
A Division of Elsevier Inc.

1600 John F. Kennedy Blvd., Suite 1800, Philadelphia, PA 19103-2899

http://www.theclinics.com

NURSING CLINICS OF NORTH AMERICA
March 2007
Editor: Ali Gavenda

Volume 42, Number 1
ISSN 0029-6465
ISBN-13: 978-1-4160-4341-6
ISBN-10: 1-4160-4341-1

The ideas and opinions expressed in *Nursing Clinics of North America* do not necessarily reflect those of the Publisher. The Publisher does not assume any responsibility for any injury and/or damage to persons or property arising out of or related to any use of the material contained in this periodical. The reader is advised to check the appropriate medical literature and the product information currently provided by the manufacturer of each drug to be administered to verify the dosage, the method and duration of administration, or contraindications. It is the responsibility of the treating physician or other health care professional, relying on independent experience and knowledge of the patient, to determine drug dosages and the best treatment for the patient. Mention of any product in this issue should not be construed as endorsement by the contributors, editors, or the Publisher of the product or manufacturers' claims.

Nursing Clinics of North America (ISSN 0029-6465) is published quarterly by Elsevier Inc., 360 Park Avenue South, New York, NY 10010-1710. Months of issue are March, June, September, and December. Business and Editorial Offices: 1600 John F. Kennedy Blvd., Suite 1800, Philadelphia, PA 19103-2899. Customer Service Office: 6277 Sea Harbor Drive, Orlando, FL 32887-4800. Periodicals postage paid at New York, NY and additional mailing offices. Subscription price per year is, $116.00 (US individuals), $216.00 (US institutions), $187.00 (international individuals), $259.00 (international institutions), $160.00 (Canadian individuals), $259.00 (Canadian institutions), $61.00 (US students), and $94.00 (international students). To receive student/resident rate, orders must be accompanied by name of affiliated institution, date of term, and the signature of program/residency coordinator on institution letterhead. Orders will be billed at individual rate until proof of status is received. Foreign air speed delivery is included in all *Clinics* subscription prices. All prices are subject to change without notice. **POSTMASTER:** Send address changes to *Nursing Clinics*, Elsevier Periodicals Customer Service, 6277 Sea Harbor Drive, Orlando, FL 32887-4800. **Customer Service: 1-800-654-2452 (US). From outside of the US, call 1-407-345-4000.**

Nursing Clinics of North America is covered in *EMBASE/Excerpta Medica, Index Medicus, Social Sciences Citation Index, Current Contents, ASCA, Cumulative Index to Nursing, RNdex Top 100*, and *Allied Health Literature and International Nursing Index (INI)*.

Printed in the United States of America.

GUEST EDITOR

JUNE HART ROMEO, PhD, NP-C, Dean and Professor, MedCentral College of Nursing, Mansfield, Ohio

CONTRIBUTORS

FREDRICK ASTLE, PhD, RNC, Assistant Professor, MedCentral College of Nursing, Mansfield, Ohio

RUTH C. McGILLIS BINDLER, RNC, PhD, Professor and Interim Associate Dean for Graduate Programs, Washington State University/Intercollegiate College of Nursing, Spokane, Washington

KATHARYN F. DAUB, EdD, CTN, CNE, RN, Associate Professor and Chair, Department of Baccalaureate Nursing, University of Hawaii at Hilo, Hilo, Hawaii

TERESA DOÑATE, MD, PhD, Servicio de Nefrologia, Fundación Puigvert, Barcelona, Spain

SANDRA FERNANDEZ, RNP, RD, Resistencia a la Insulina SL, Barcelona, Spain

PAUL HYMAN, PhD, Associate Professor, MedCentral College of Nursing, Mansfield, Ohio

JERONI JURADO, RN, DNS, Primary Care, Catalan Health Institute, Olot (Girona), Spain

PAUL KELNER, MD, Associate Professor and Director of Science, MedCentral College of Nursing, Mansfield, Ohio

JULIE MILLER, RN, MSN, Assistance Professor, MedCentral College of Nursing, Mansfield, Ohio

ANTONIO PÉREZ, MD, PhD, Departamento de Medicina, Universitat Autònoma de Barcelona, Barcelona, Spain

JOSEP MARIA POU, MD, PhD, Servicio de Endocrinología y Nutrición, Hospital de Sant Pau, Barcelona, Spain

GINGER RATERINK, DNSC, ANP-C, Assistant Professor, Department of Nursing, University of Colorado Health Sciences Center, Denver, Colorado

JUNE HART ROMEO, PhD, NP-C, Dean and Professor, MedCentral College of Nursing, Mansfield, Ohio

JOAN SÁNCHEZ-HERNÁNDEZ, MD, PhD, Servicio de Endocrinología y Nutrición, Hospital de Sant Pau; and Departamento de Medicina, Universitat Autónoma de Barcelona, Barcelona, Spain

JUAN YBARRA, MD, PhD, FACE, Servicio de Endocrinología y Nutrición, Hospital de Sant Pau; and Instituto de Cardiología Avanzada y Medicina, Centro Médico Teknon, Barcelona, Spain

CONTENTS

positive and negative predictive values. The predicted probability of DPN diagnosis was higher with tuning fork evaluation.

Diabetes and Depression: A Review of the Literature 67
Fredrick Astle

Depression affects millions of people in the United States. Drugs used to treat depression can lead to weight gain, which could predispose a person to type 2 diabetes. Also, certain medications that may be used to treat depression with psychotic features can lead to metabolic syndrome and new-onset diabetes. Diabetes is another chronic health care condition that affects millions of people in the United States. Diabetes is the leading cause of nontraumatic amputations and a leading cause of blindness. Both conditions can result in a lower quality of life. Clinicians face challenges in treating either condition, but can face greater ones when the conditions occur together. This article reviews the literature concerning depression and diabetes.

Primary Hyperparathyroidism, Insulin Resistance, and Cardiovascular Disease: A Review 79
Juan Ybarra, Teresa Doñate, Jeroni Jurado, and Josep Maria Pou

The presentation of primary hyperparathyroidism (PHPT) has changed substantially in the last decade. Before the introduction of routine calcium measurement in most automated biochemistry serum analyzers, it usually was diagnosed after renal and bony lesions already were present. Nowadays, its presentation is practically asymptomatic. Nevertheless, the cardiovascular morbidity and mortality of mild to moderate forms of PHPT reportedly are increasing. Individuals who have mild to moderate forms of PHPT have an increased risk for enduring cardiovascular disease, arterial hypertension, left ventricular hypertrophy, myocardial and valvular calcifications, altered vascular reactivity, and cardiac conduction. Finally, they also reveal alterations in carbohydrate metabolism, insulin resistance, dyslipidemia, and body composition.

Hypogonadal Hypogonadism and Osteoporosis in Men 87
June Hart Romeo and Juan Ybarra

In recent years, osteoporosis in men has become increasingly recognized as an important clinical and public health problem. Many similarities exist in various aspects of osteoporosis in men and women, but this article focuses on the sex difference, bone biology, epidemiology, and consequences of fractures. Although maintenance of bone integrity depends on the action of sex hormones in both sexes, menopause is a much more obvious indicator of estrogen deficiency than is the subtle decrease of testosterone in aging men. This often leads to delay and neglect of diagnosis. The need to identify and screen men at particular risk for osteoporosis, as when hypogonadism is induced for treatment of prostate cancer, has become important.

Pheochromocytomas are catecholamine-secreting tumors arising from chromaffin cells of the sympathoadrenal system, which includes the adrenal medulla and sympathetic ganglionic tissue. The effects of catecholamine excess cause potentially fatal symptomologies and end-organ damage if not diagnosed and treated. If diagnosed and removed surgically, most of these patients can be cured. Pheochromocytomas are rare and affect from two to eight per million people. There are 800 deaths in the United States annually as a result of complications. Of patients who have pheochromocytomas diagnosed at autopsy, 75% died suddenly from myocardial infarction or cerebral vascular catastrophe. Challenges in diagnosis, tumor location, and treatment are considerable.

A primary goal of nurses providing care for persons who have diabetes mellitus or thyroid disease is improving their health outcomes. For persons who have diabetes and thyroid disease and live in poverty, improving the care process, and ultimately health outcomes, must include the nurse's understanding of poverty. The purpose of this article is to provide nurses with a basic understanding of the resource issues, "hidden rules," and characteristics that are associated with persons who live in poverty. Most importantly, some basic strategies to improve the health outcomes of patients who have diabetes or thyroid disease and live in poverty are provided.

Dehydration commonly leads to hypovolemia and hemoconcentration. Changes in thyroid hormone–binding proteins secondary to hemoconcentration profoundly affect total serum thyroid hormone concentrations. The authors sought to determine the acute effects of mild to moderate dehydration on thyroid hormone levels/thyroid function tests and its reversibility upon rehydration.

Total thyroxine, total triiodothyronine, free thyroxine, and the free-thyroxine index decreased significantly after hydration, in parallel with the decrease in extracellular fluid volume status markers. Triiodothyronine-resin uptake increased after hydration. Thyrotropin levels decreased by 8% after hydration. Hypovolemia leads to simultaneous alterations in extracellular fluid volume markers and thyroid hormone serum concentrations that reverse rapidly upon rehydration. This constitutes, by itself, a distinct and new clinical entity.

FORTHCOMING ISSUES

RECENT ISSUES

THE CLINICS ARE NOW AVAILABLE ONLINE!

Access your subscription at:
http://www.theclinics.com

ELSEVIER
SAUNDERS

Nurs Clin N Am 42 (2007) xi–xii

NURSING
CLINICS
OF NORTH AMERICA

Preface

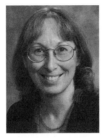

June Hart Romeo, PhD, NP-C
Guest Editor

One of the wonderful things about being a nurse is the constant challenge and excitement in our evolving profession. Although the spirit of caring has been the mainstay of nursing for decades, it is no longer enough. Today's nurse is intellectually capable of synthesizing hundreds of bits of data to come up with an appropriate plan of care, has enough political savvy to negotiate the most convoluted health care system, and is able to apply research findings into an evidence-based practice, all while maintaining a core of compassion for patients and their families.

Nowhere is all this more evident than in endocrine nursing. Endocrine nursing requires a strong intellect and an ability to solve problems. It requires the nurse to be able to take a myriad of seemingly unrelated pieces of data from a patient's history, physical assessment, and laboratory and diagnostic test reports, and make sense out of it. It requires the nurse to have cutting-edge knowledge as the foundation for professional practice.

In this issue of the *Nursing Clinics of North America*, we have put together a collection of articles based on the most up-to-date information available. Nurses, physicians, and scientists share information that will help strengthen their practice. It has been exciting for me to begin a dialog with

doi:10.1016/j.cnur.2006.12.002   *nursing.theclinics.com* our authors, and I hope our readers, too, will find this issue stimulating and thought-provoking.

June Hart Romeo, PhD, NP-C
MedCentral College of Nursing
335 Glessner Avenue
Mansfield, OH 44903, USA

E-mail address: jromeo@medcentral.edu

ELSEVIER
SAUNDERS

NURSING
CLINICS
OF NORTH AMERICA

Nurs Clin N Am 42 (2007) 1–18

Pharmacotherapeutic Uses of Hormones

Paul Hyman, PhD*, Paul Kelner, MD

MedCentral College of Nursing, 335 Glessner Avenue, Mansfield, OH 44903, USA

The use of hormones as pharmacotherapeutic agents falls into two broad categories: restoration of missing (or decreased) hormones to normal levels and augmentation to supraphysiologic levels. Arguably, the former can trace its roots to the earliest use of animal gland extracts to counter the (then unknown) effects of aging, whereas the latter requires the greater understanding of human biology and hormone activity gained in recent times. This understanding now places hormones firmly in the modern apothecary. For many purposes, there is little difference between the use of hormones and other types of drugs; however, their biologic origins do present particular advantages and disadvantages (eg, in terms of synthesis, mode of administration).

This article reviews the biology of the various classes of hormones. It then reviews some of the more common diseases that are treated with hormones (or analogs); this section is not exhaustive because of space limitations, but many of the most commonly used hormones are described. Finally, some trends in the future development of hormone-related drugs are described.

A note about references: because much of the information reviewed in this paper is standard, references are limited to those dealing with new information or harder to find background information. In preparing this review, the authors relied on Richard A. Lehne's *Pharmacology for Nursing Care* [1], but most other current pharmacology texts have similar information. We also found that the Wikipedia on the Internet is an excellent source of historical and other background information about many drugs and related conditions [2].

The biology of hormones

A hormone can be defined as "a substance that originates in an organ, gland or part and is conveyed through the blood to another part of the

* Corresponding author.
E-mail address: phyman@medcentral.edu (P. Hyman).

doi:10.1016/j.cnur.2006.11.002

body, stimulating it by chemical action to increase functional activity or to increase secretion of another hormone" [3]. A simpler, if less precise, definition is that hormones are chemical messengers that are carried in the bloodstream from their site of production to their targets. Chemically, hormones are traditionally divided into two groups: steroids and peptides. Steroid hormones are lipids, derived from cholesterol, and all share a common steroid carbon skeleton. Peptide hormones include modified amino acids, small peptides, and larger proteins. In recent years, a third class of hormones has been identified, the eicosanoids. These lipid hormones are derived from a fatty acid, arachidonic acid.

Hormones are produced mainly by endocrine glands, ductless glands that release their hormone products directly into the bloodstream; however a few hormones are produced by other tissues, including the heart, kidneys, adipose cells, and the placenta.

Steroids

Steroid hormones all have a four-carbon ring skeleton and differ in the chemical groups that are attached to this common "backbone." They all are derived from cholesterol and are produced principally by cells in the adrenal cortex and the gonads. The steroids that are produced by the adrenal cortex are collectively referred to as corticosteroids. They include more than a dozen different hormones, although the bulk of the corticosteroids consist of two main families: the glucocorticoids, which help to regulate metabolism, and the mineralocorticoids, which regulate serum salt levels and fluid balance within the body. The other major group of steroids is the sex hormones, which are produced principally by the gonads (ovaries and testes), although small amounts are made by other tissues throughout the body. Sex hormones are divided into the androgens (eg, testosterone) and estrogens (eg, estradiol). Androgens and estrogens are produced by men and women, although the relative amounts are different in each gender. The sex hormones are associated with the development of the reproductive tract, gamete production, and maintenance of secondary sexual characteristics.

Peptide hormones

Peptide hormones form a chemically more varied group of molecules than do the steroid hormones. Peptide hormones range in size from modified single amino acids to the 191–amino acid growth hormone protein. A few peptide hormones are modified by the addition of otherwise inorganic atoms. For example, the thyroid hormones require iodine to be active, the major use of iodine in human metabolism. Unlike steroid hormones that usually are made as needed, peptide hormones often are made by cells and stored in an inactive (prohormone) form until needed. This allows for the release of large amounts of peptide hormones when they are needed. Physiologically, peptide hormones often are involved in controlling many of the homeostatic mechanisms of the body, and may affect many different target cell types or only a few. Peptide hormones are produced by all of the glands that compose the endocrine system as well as other tissues. The major peptide hormone–producing glands are the hypothalamus, pituitary gland, pineal gland, thyroid and parathyroid glands, thymus, adrenal gland, pancreas, and gonads. In addition, cells within the heart, kidneys, adipose tissue, and placenta produce peptide hormones. Despite the large number of peptide hormone–producing tissues, each peptide hormone is produced by a single cell type within a single gland or tissue.

Eicosanoids

The eicosanoids are derived from the 20-carbon fatty acid arachidonic acid, and, hence, represent an additional chemical class of hormones. Eicosanoids tend to act locally, and, thus, are not classic circulating hormones; however, they share most other characteristics with hormones and so are beginning to be classified with them. There are two main groups of eicosanoids: the leukotrienes and the prostaglandins. Leukotrienes mediate some immune responses, especially those involved in allergic reactions. They also are mediators of inflammation. Through both of these mechanisms, the leukotrienes have a critical role in diseases such as asthma. Prostaglandins have a wider range of affects. Effects of prostaglandins include triggering muscle contractions in the uterus during childbirth; inducing vasoconstriction or vasodilation, and, thus, affecting blood pressure; enhancing platelet aggregation, and, hence, blood clotting; regulating renal blood flow and gastric mucosa activity; and mediating inflammation.

Other molecules

There are other signaling molecules within the body that do not completely fit the traditional definitions of hormones. Most segments of the digestive tract produce peptides that act in nearby segments to regulate the movement of materials through the digestive tract. Because these paracrine hormones do not enter the general circulation, some sources exclude them as hormones, but otherwise, they seem to act like other hormones. Likewise, angiogenesis factors (that promote blood vessel growth) and other cell growth factors and inhibitors can be considered as peptide hormones by some definitions. Further complicating a simple classification of molecules as hormones or not, some neurotransmitters, such as epinephrine and norepinephrine, are chemically identical to adrenaline and noradrenaline, respectively. Finally, the gas nitric oxide (NO) acts as a signaling molecule as well as a neurotransmitter. In blood vessels, NO is a potent vasodilator; this activity is behind the mechanism of action of nitroglycerin in relieving symptoms of angina by relaxing and opening partially occluded coronary vessels. This vasodilation and other effects of NO on the circulatory system also are behind the circulatory collapse that is associated with bacterial sepsis when macrophages produce excess NO as part of their bacteria-killing mechanism [4].

Hormone receptors

Because hormones circulate throughout the body, each hormone molecule can have the potential to interact with nearly any cell. Although some hormones, such as insulin, thyroid hormones, and growth hormone, have an effect on many different types of cells, others, such as erythropoietin and the releasing hormones produced by the hypothalamus, are highly specific in their effects. The cells that are affected by a hormone are referred to as the hormone's target cells. For a hormone to affect a target cell, the cell must make a receptor protein that binds the hormone. It is the receptor proteins, rather than any feature of the hormone itself, that determine which cells are the target cells of the hormone. The receptors for peptide hormones are almost always membrane proteins. Steroid hormone receptors usually are found in the target cell's cytoplasm or nucleus, because steroid hormones are lipids that can pass through the cell membrane. These different locations reflect the differing mechanisms of hormone action that are seen commonly with peptide and steroid hormones.

A peptide hormone binding to its receptor typically triggers a cascade of signal molecules within the cell. The first of these signal molecules often are described as second messengers (the peptide hormone being the first messenger), and they are produced by proteins called G-proteins. In fact, the receptor proteins sometimes are referred to as G-protein–coupled receptors; these receptors, along with the G-proteins, represent new targets for drug discovery research [5]. The effect of the production of the second messengers depends on the specific molecule as well as the cell type. The cell may respond in many ways, such as changing its membrane permeability to particular molecules (eg, kidney nephron cells adjust their rate of Ca^{2+} readsorption in response to parathyroid hormone [PTH]), releasing stored substances (eg, mammary gland cells releasing milk in response to oxytocin), and contracting (eg, vasoconstriction of the peripheral circulatory vessels in response to adrenaline). The production of second messengers, also referred to as signal transduction, allows the target cells to integrate signals from multiple hormones and other cell conditions, which lets the body fine-tune the responses of various tissues and organs.

Unlike the peptide receptors, steroid receptors typically are located within the cell. The effect of a steroid hormone binding to its receptor is also usually different from that of peptide hormones. Typically, the receptor protein is a DNA-binding protein that usually requires the bound hormone to bind to DNA. The receptor–hormone complex may activate or inactivate expression of a particular set of genes. For example, aldosterone causes the kidney's nephron cells to alter expression of several ion transport proteins to increase readsorption of Na^+ and water; therefore, it affects ion and water balance, and, indirectly, blood pressure. Because steroid hormones typically affect the protein expression profile of the target tissues, steroid hormone effects are not as rapid as are those of peptide hormones, but they can be much longer lasting.

The eicosanoids—although they are lipids like the steroid hormones—bind to membrane receptors and exert their effects through second messengers like most peptide hormones [6].

Using hormones as pharmacologic agents

Hormones are used in the pharmacotherapeutic arena for conditions that fall into two main categories: conditions that arise from subnormal levels of a particular hormone as part of disease or as a result of aging, and conditions where supranormal levels of a hormone confer some benefit on the patient. We present several examples of each and of drugs that act as hormone antagonists. Lastly, we briefly examine two examples of the abuse of hormones for nontherapeutic purposes.

Insulin for the treatment of diabetes (type 1)

Although diabetes (more properly, diabetes mellitus) was described (and named) by the ancient Greeks, its mechanism was only identified definitively in the beginning of the twentieth century. In the early 1920s, the first isolation of insulin and its use as a treatment for diabetes was demonstrated using bovine insulin. It was only later that the difference between type 1 and type 2 diabetes was made clear. More recently has come the recognition that type 1 diabetes is usually caused by an autoimmune response against the β-islet cells in the pancreas that secrete insulin.

The isolation of insulin quickly led to its use as a treatment for diabetes. For many years, only animal sources of insulin were available in quantity. Because bovine and porcine insulin are nearly identical to human insulin, they supplied an effective substitute although problems with contaminating proteins remained. In the 1980s, several companies developed recombinant forms of insulin using the human gene expressed in bacteria from which purer preparations could be made. Currently, a variety of human insulins are available. Some are identical to the human protein, whereas others are insulin analogs that have been modified to be absorbed more quickly (Aspart and Lispro) or for greater stability within the body (Detemir and Glargine).

In the treatment of type 1 diabetes, insulin replacement is only part of a complete treatment regimen. Control of diet, exercise, and regular monitoring of blood glucose levels must be accomplished in addition to the taking of insulin. Because insulin is a protein that would be digested if taken orally (although research into oral forms of insulin is being done), insulin is usually injected with needle and syringe by the patient one or more times per day. Other modes of administration of insulin include pen injectors, insulin pumps (external or internal), and jet injection. In January 2006, the U.S. Food and Drug Administration (FDA) announced approval of the first inhaled form of insulin, which is expected to be on the market sometime in 2006 [7].

The mode and timing of injections depends on the abilities of the patient, the patient's age, activity level, overall health, and diet. For example, growth during adolescence and infection at any age indicate a need for an increase in insulin dosage, whereas exercise usually decreases the need for insulin. Different types of insulin also demand different dosing schedules and injection sites. For example, fast-acting short-duration insulin analogs (eg, Lispro or Aspart insulins) can be injected just before or after meals, whereas long-acting analogs (eg, Glargine insulin) normally are injected only once per day. Generally, fast-acting insulins are injected into the abdominal muscle, whereas longer-lasting forms are injected into the arm or leg. Because diabetics require insulin daily for their entire lives, the patients must take an especially active role in determining their dosage of insulin.

Growth hormone for the treatment of dwarfism

Human growth hormone (to differentiate it from the animal proteins in widespread commercial use in agriculture) or hGH is also called somatotropin. It is produced by the anterior pituitary gland in response to growth hormone–releasing hormone from the hypothalamus. Growth hormone promotes the growth of muscle and bone as well as other organ systems (especially in childhood). In exerting these growth effects, hGH also affects cellular metabolism, which leads to an increase in protein synthesis and carbohydrate use. A lack of hGH in children leads to a failure to grow or dwarfism. The effects in adults are less obvious, appearing as a slow decrease in muscle and bone mass that often is associated with decreased energy levels. Not all cases of children lagging in growth are due to a lack of growth hormone, and the patient's growth hormone levels should be determined before any treatment with growth hormone. There are also forms of dwarfism (eg, achondroplasia, campomelic dysplasia, spondyloepiphyseal dysplasia) that are not due to a lack of hGH. In addition to treating dwarfism that is due to hGH deficiency, hGH is approved to treat somatotropin deficiency in adults, shortness in children due to chronic renal insufficiency or Turner's syndrome, and cachexia in patients who have AIDS.

First isolated from cadaver pituitary glands in the 1950s, hGH was a scarce and highly priced drug until the gene was cloned successfully in the early 1980s. The recombinant form of the hormone (rhGH) quickly replaced the isolated protein because of availability and because it removed the specter of iatrogenic disease, specifically Creutzfeld-Jacob disease. Nevertheless, hGH remained and remains costly. In addition to cost and availability, several ethical issues still surround the use of hGH and rhGH treatment for nonlife-threatening conditions. A good overview of the history and controversies can be found online [8]. The use of hGH as an "antiaging" medication is discussed later.

There are two different forms of rhGH available: somatrem (Protropin), which differs from hGH by one amino acid, and somatropin (many brands), which is identical to hGH. Both are approved for treating dwarfism in children, whereas somatropin is approved for treating the other conditions listed above. As a drug, both forms are injected subcutaneously or intramuscularly as fresh preparations of a reconstituted powder. Patients receive a dose based on body weight, and usually receive three to seven injections per week. Usually, treatment is continued throughout childhood until growth stops in the late teens. It is important to monitor epiphyseal growth in the long bones so that treatment can be stopped to allow epiphyseal fusion at the end of growth.

For children whose growth is retarded for reasons other than a lack of hGH, treatment with hGH has limited effect, and its use remains controversial, often depending on psychologic factors [9,10].

Thyroid hormones for the treatment of hypothyroidism

In response to thyrotropin, produced by the pituitary gland, the thyroid gland produces and releases two hormones: thyroxine (T_4) and triiodothyronine (T_3). T_3 and T_4 are nearly identical and differ only in the number of iodine atoms that they contain; many cell are able to convert T_4 into T_3. Together, these two hormones have a profound effect on many cell types, including a general stimulation of basal cellular metabolism (resulting in increased use of oxygen and heat production) and significant growth stimulation during childhood. A lack of thyroid hormones (hypothyroidism) can have profound effects in childhood, especially in infants, leading to mental retardation and failure of growth in many organ systems (cretinism). In adults, symptoms are related to a lowered metabolism and include fatigue, lethargy, decreased body temperature and heart rate, dry skin, and hair loss. Depending on the underlying cause, a goiter may or may not develop.

Hypothyroidism may arise in several ways, including autoimmune attack on the thyroid, physical damage to the thyroid, or iatrogenic effects from treatment of depression or cancer. Initially, hypothyroidism was treated with thyroid hormones derived from pig thyroids. Unlike most hormones, thyroid hormones can be absorbed effectively by the digestive tract so they can be administered orally. In the 1950s, synthetic thyroid hormones became available. Today, patients may take synthetic hormones (levothyroxine [T_4], liothyronine [T_3], or liotrix [a mix of T_3 and T_4]) or a purified extract from animal thyroid glands. Because many cells in the body can convert the T_4 hormone into the T_3 hormone, it is not uncommon for a patient to take only the T_4 hormone; however, the efficiency of conversion varies between individuals as well as between tissues in the body, which causes a subset of patients to respond poorly to T_4 alone. For these patients, a mix of T_4 and T_3 results in a better overall prognosis [11].

Hormone replacement therapy with estrogens and progestins

Estrogens and progesterone are steroid hormones that are produced principally by the ovarian follicular and luteal cells and secondarily by the adrenal cortex in women. They play critical roles in the reproductive cycles of women and in pregnancy. As drugs, estrogens and progestins (synthetic analogs of progesterone) have two major uses: in contraceptives and as replacement hormones after menopause (or hysterectomy or ovariectomy). Here, the discussion is limited to hormone replacement therapy (HRT).

Menopause is a normal part of the aging process for women, occurring as the ovaries decrease and then cease normal ovulatory cycling. The decrease and cessation of estrogen production has effects on multiple organ systems in addition to the reproductive system.

> Loss of estrogen has multiple consequences. Prominent among these are vasomotor symptoms (manifesting as hot flushes, also known as hot flashes, and night sweats), urogenital atrophy (manifesting as vaginal dryness, itching, and burning), and accelerated bone loss (manifesting as osteoporosis and fractures) [1].

HRT, using estrogens alone or estrogens plus progestins (which are added to counter the growth stimulatory effects of estrogens on the uterus that might promote uterine cancer), have been used to alleviate some or all of these symptoms. Some early data also indicated a potential protective effect against heart disease. This early data, along with many other questions, led the National Institutes of Health (NIH) to include heart disease in the Women's Health Initiative (WHI). Begun in 1991, the WHI recruited women to participate in a series of clinical trials and observational studies on HRT and two other preventive treatment strategies. Although ongoing, intermediate results of these studies and others (eg, the Heart and Estrogen/Progestin Replacement Study [HERS]) have already led to major changes in the use of HRT. It is now clear that HRT is a treatment with specific risks that must be balanced against the benefits of relieving menopausal symptoms. Whether in the form of estrogen plus progestin or estrogen alone, HRT must be tailored to the particular needs of the patient and reassessed frequently to ensure a favorable risk/benefit ratio. Because results of ongoing studies are being released even as this review was being written, we recommend that interested readers consult the FDA and NIH Web sites for the latest information [12,13].

In addition to postmenopausal-related symptoms and heart disease, estrogens and progestins have been shown to affect rates of cancer of the reproductive organs, breast, and colon. For some women, HRT increases the risk, but for others it seems to have a protective effect. This depends, in part, on the specific type of HRT being administered. For example, short-term estrogen plus progestin treatment increases the overall risk for breast cancer in postmenopausal women [14], but estrogen-only (using conjugated equine estrogen) treatment seems not to increase this risk and may be slightly protective [15]. Conversely, estrogen plus progestin is protective against the development of colon cancer. As with other results of the WHI studies, the data on cancer is still being developed and analyzed. The latest results and links to the most recent publications are available on the WHI Web site [16].

Parathyroid hormone and calcitonin in the treatment of calcium imbalances and osteoporosis

These two polypeptide hormones make up an antagonistic pair to control serum calcium levels. PTH is released by the parathyroid glands in response to low plasma calcium levels. PTH affects the kidneys where it increases rates of vitamin D activation and calcium readsorption; the intestinal tract, where it increase rates of calcium adsorption; and the bones, where osteoclast cells are stimulated to release calcium into the blood (bone resorption). In contrast, calcitonin is released by the parafollicular cells of the thyroid gland in response to elevated plasma calcium. Calcitonin inhibits osteoclast resorption of bone and promotes the incorporation of calcium into the mineral matrix of bone. Pharmacologically, a recombinant analog of PTH (teriparatide), which contains the first 34 amino acids of the native 84 residue peptide, is indicated for use in women who have osteoporosis and are at significant risk for fracture. It is generally recommended for women who have not responded well to calcium/vitamin D supplementation or to bisphosphates (inhibitors of bone resorption). Unlike these other drugs for osteoporosis that act by inhibiting bone resorption, teriparatide increases bone formation. It is generally given by daily injection. This is similar to native PTH, which can increase bone density when given in daily injections so that PTH levels increase transiently [1].

Calcitonin is available as a subcutaneous or intramuscular injection and as a nasal spray. The drug form of calcitonin used most commonly is calcitonin-salmon, which is extracted from salmon. It is more potent than human calcitonin on a per weight basis. Pharmacologic indications for calcitonin include the treatment of Paget's disease of bone (osteitis deformans), hypercalcemia, and osteoporosis.

Glucagon for treatment of hypoglycemia

Glucagon is a 29–amino acid polypeptide hormone that is synthesized by the α-cells found in the islets of Langerhans of the pancreas. It is released in response to serum hypoglycemia, and it increases serum glucose by inducing glycogenolysis in the liver. It also acts to relax the smooth muscle of the gastrointestinal tract. Glucagon is prepared for pharmacologic use by recombinant DNA technology. Its major clinical uses include the treatment of acute hypoglycemia that is due to insulin overdose (especially if glucose cannot be given by mouth or parenterally), and as an adjunct in radiographic imaging of the gastrointestinal tract. Glucagon also has shown efficacy in the treatment of overdose that is due to β-blockers or calcium channel blockers.

Antidiuretic hormone as a vasoconstrictor and in the treatment of nocturnal enuresis

Antidiuretic hormone (ADH) is a nine–amino acid hormone that is produced in the neurosecretory cells of the hypothalamus and stored in the posterior pituitary. It is released in response to elevated serum osmolality. The primary physiologic action of ADH is to increase the permeability of the nephronal collecting ducts to water, which leads to reabsorption of water back into the circulation, increased blood volume, and decreased osmolality. ADH also is referred to as vasopressin, because its presence results in constriction of vascular and gastrointestinal smooth muscle cells. These actions, coupled with its role in water balance, make ADH useful in the hormone-derived pharmacologic armamentarium.

ADH is commercially available as desmopressin (a modified form of human ADH) and vasopressin (which is identical to human ADH). Desmopressin is indicated for treatment of polyuria/polydipsia associated with diabetes insipidus (excessive urine production not associated with diabetes mellitus), primary nocturnal enuresis (bedwetting), and spontaneous or traumatic bleeding in patients who have hemophilia A or von Willebrand disease. The primary labeled indication for vasopressin also is in diabetes insipidus, but it also is used as part of the Advanced Cardiac Life Support protocol as an alternative to, or in conjunction with, epinephrine in the treatment of ventricular fibrillation, pulseless electrical activity, and asystole [17]. In this situation, it seems that vasopressin increases tissue perfusion in the heart, especially in the case of asystole. Vasopressin is also effective in treating some cases of gastrointestinal hemorrhage, such as ruptured esophageal varices.

Growth hormone supplementation as an "antiaging" therapy

hGH, whose production normally declines with age, often is promoted as being able to reduce several physical changes that are associated with aging, such as decreased muscle mass, strength, and endurance. Many of the claims can be traced back to a preliminary study by Rudman and colleagues [18] that was published in 1990. A few of the results have been confirmed; however, many of the other claims that have been made for hGH have been shown to be wrong, and potential risks of hGH treatment of adults have been identified (see Refs. [19,20] for an overview). Still an "antiaging" industry has developed around the sale of hGH and hGH stimulants as dietary supplements. There have been no reputable scientific studies to support this use, and the FDA has specifically disallowed this use of hGH [20].

We now turn to several examples of the use of hormones at supranormal levels to achieve a therapeutic effect. These include recognized and experimental treatments.

Somatostatin in the treatment of acromegaly and gigantism

Acromegaly in adults and gigantism (giantism) in children are the result of an overproduction of hGH. This overproduction may be due to a problem in the pituitary gland, which makes growth hormone, or in the hypothalamus gland, which produces growth hormone–releasing factor (GHRF) and growth hormone–inhibiting factor (GHIF or somatostatin), the primary controls on growth hormone synthesis and release. Overproduction of GHRF, underproduction of somatostatin, or overproduction of hGH directly can lead to acromegaly or gigantism. Both conditions have common features of excessive growth in bones, joints, and muscles leading to overlarge hands and feet and a characteristic large jaw. The major difference is that patients who have gigantism have above average height, whereas those who suffer from acromegaly will not, because the epiphyseal growth plates in the long bones are fused before the onset of the disease.

For some patients, an increase in somatostatin levels is sufficient to bring hGH levels back to normal. Native somatostatin is a two-chain polypeptide of 14 and 28 amino acids; however, an eight-residue peptide analog of somatostatin (Octreotide) has been found to be equally effective at downregulating hGH production. Like other peptide hormones, it must be injected. Often, it is used in conjunction with surgical or radiation ablation of the pituitary.

Glucocorticoids

Glucocorticoids are a class of steroid hormones. Produced by the cortex of the adrenal glands, their primary physiologic role is the regulation of energy metabolism. The principal glucocorticoid is cortisol, and, along with the other glucocorticoids, it is released by the adrenal glands throughout the day as part of the homeostatic mechanism for maintaining glucose levels in the blood. In addition, the glucocorticoids play a role in fluid balance within the body and are produced in response to stress, which lead to increased levels of fat, protein, and carbohydrate metabolism, presumably as a part of general protective mechanisms.

Damage to the adrenal cortex (ie, Addison's disease) or other causes can lead to insufficient production of glucocorticoids. In these cases, glucocorticoids (and other adrenal corticosteroids or analogs) are given in physiologic doses. Glucocorticoids also are given at times when the patient may be under excessive stress, such as surgery [21]; however, these uses of glucocorticoids are not the major uses of these hormones as drugs. At high doses, glucocorticoids are potent inhibitors of inflammation and immune cell growth. The mechanism by which this occurs is not completely understood, but it seems to be multifactorial and involves the down-regulation of a series of cytokine genes as well as the up-regulation of several hormone receptors [22]. This activity allows the glucocorticoids (commonly, if not correctly, referred to as corticosteroids in this context) to be used to treat various inflammatory disorders (eg, asthma, inflammatory bowel diseases, rheumatoid arthritis), as well as part of immunosuppressive therapy for transplants and some autoimmune diseases. They also are used to treat some lymphatic system cancers.

Cortisol (hydrocortisone) and its synthetic analogs are used for various glucocorticoid applications. Because these are all steroids that can pass through cell membranes, they can be administered in a variety of ways, depending on whether systemic or local treatment is needed. Local therapy, including inhaled, topical, and injected (eg, into a joint) applications, minimizes the therapeutic dosage and systemic effects. It should be remembered, however, that some systemic absorption will occur even after local administration, because even local applications are large compared with normal physiologic doses of glucocorticoids. When systemic therapy is needed, oral administration generally provides a better drug dissemination than does injection. For several particular analogs, intravenous administration is preferred for systemic therapy.

Some of the analogs, as well as hydrocortisone, also act as mineralocorticoids when given at pharmacologic dosages. This means that they can alter the body's mineral and fluid balance and lead to water and sodium retention and potassium loss. The high doses also can inhibit production of corticosteroids by the adrenal glands as well as result in other, more specific, side effects. When immunosuppression is not the therapeutic goal, immunosuppression also can be considered an undesirable side effect. It is important, therefore, to monitor patients closely and to determine dosages empirically for each patient. Ideally, patients start with low doses that are increased until symptom relief is obtained. Glucocorticoids also should be withdrawn slowly to allow the body to adapt to producing its own glucocorticoids again.

Lastly, in addition to their direct use in the chemotherapy of lymphatic cancers, such as Hodgkin's disease, glucocorticoids are used as an adjunct to chemotherapy of other cancers. In this role, they are used to reduce pain, suppress nausea and vomiting, limit radiation-induced edema, and provide other symptom relief.

Hormone treatments of cancer

In addition to the glucocorticoids, other hormones or their analogs are used in the treatment of specific neoplasms. Many new cancer treatments are in, or are emerging from, clinical trials; it is likely that many new treatments will be added to this category.

Prostate cancer may be treated using analogs of gonadotropin-releasing hormone (GnRH). These drugs (leuprolide, triptorelin, goserelin) lead to a down-regulation of androgens (mainly testosterone). Because most prostate cancer cells are androgen dependent, this slows the growth of the cancer. GnRH analogs are sometimes given in conjunction with one of another set of drugs that blocks the androgen receptor. Androgen receptor antagonists (flutamide, bicalutamide, or nilutamide) enhance the activity of the GnRH analogs by blocking the activity of androgens that are produced in tissues unaffected by the GnRH mimics. In addition, estrogens, which also inhibit androgen production, may be used.

Androgens and progestins are used sometimes to treat some breast cancers that have proven resistant to antiestrogen compounds and other first-line chemotherapeutic agents. Because not all breast cancer cells make the progesterone receptor, tumors should be screened to see if progestin treatment is a viable option.

Renal carcinomas may be treated with interleukin (IL)-2, a peptide stimulant of the immune system. (Although the interleukins sometimes are not considered to be hormones because a defined gland does not produce them, they do circulate and affect cells at a distance from the cells that produce them.) A recombinant IL-2 (aldesleukin) has been approved for treating metastatic renal cancer, and it is being studied for the treatment of other cancers. It is likely that IL-2 does not affect the cancer cells directly, but rather alters the patient's immune response against the tumor cells. Other interleukins are also being studied as cancer immunotherapeutic agents [23].

Some cancers are not treated with hormones or hormone analogs, but with compounds that are antagonistic to particular hormones. These include antiandrogens and antiestrogens. The antiandrogens are the androgen receptor antagonists mentioned above that are often used in conjunction with the GnRH analogs. Antiestrogens include fulvestrant, tamoxifen, and toremifene. The latter two also are described as selective estrogen receptor modulators (SERMs), because they block an estrogen receptor in some tissues and activate a receptor in others. This occurs, in part, because cells in different tissues make differing amounts of three different estrogen receptors. Fulvestrant only interferes with estrogen receptor activation. All three antiestrogens are used to treat breast cancers that depend on estrogens for efficient growth (estrogen receptor-positive breast cancers). The two SERMs also have been studied as breast cancer preventive agents. Unfortunately, tamoxifen use increases a woman's risk for endometrial cancer because of the compound's stimulatory effects on uterine cells. Toremifene is known to stimulate uterine cell hyperplasia, but the risk for uterine cancer is not known. Other antiestrogens are in development or in clinical trials.

A separate class of antiestrogens is the aromatase inhibitors (anastrozole, letrozole, exemestane) that block the conversion of androgens into estrogens. These drugs target estrogen synthesis outside of the ovary only, so their use is limited to postmenopausal women who have breast cancer. Clinical trials to compare the aromatase inhibitors with tamoxifen for efficacy alone and in combination are underway.

Leukotriene antagonists in the treatment of asthma

Among the newer drugs that are used for the treatment of asthma are those that interfere with the actions of the eicosanoid leukotrienes. Leukotrienes trigger bronchoconstriction, inflammation, and recruitment of immune cells into the bronchioles, among other effects. By blocking these functions, they alleviate many of the symptoms of asthma. Three leukotriene inhibitors are in use. One (zileuton) prevents leukotriene synthesis, whereas the other two (zafirlukast and montelukast) act as leukotriene receptor blockers. Unlike many (but not all) asthma drugs, all three of the leukotriene inhibitors are taken orally, and, hence, are delivered systemically. Because all three are new, the best way to integrate their use into existing drug protocols for the management of asthma is still being developed.

Hormone abuse: anabolic steroids and erythropoietin

Androgens (in this context usually referred to as anabolic steroids or merely steroids) have been used in a nontherapeutic context for many years by athletes for increasing muscle growth and performance enhancement. Unlike some of the "dietary supplements" that have been demonstrated to have little efficacy (eg, androstenedione [Andro]) [24], controlled studies have shown that this use of androgens can be efficacious when given in sufficiently high doses [25]. Nevertheless, this use of androgens is considered abuse because there is no pathologic condition being treated, and the risk for adverse effects is significant. Androgen abuse can be associated with fluid and salt imbalance that leads to hypertension, increased LDL and decreased HDL, and liver toxicity, among other adverse effects. Adult women also may suffer menstrual irregularities and virilization—the development of secondary male sexual characteristics, such as facial hair and deepening voice—as well as uterine and breast atrophy. Often, some virilization effects are permanent, even when androgen use is stopped. Adult men may have suppression of luteinizing hormone and follicle-stimulating hormone, which lead to decreased sperm development, testicular atrophy, and consequent sterility, as well as gynecomastia (breast development). In boys and girls who have not finished normal growth, androgens can lead to stunted growth by triggering premature epiphyseal closure in the long bones.

Given these serious adverse effects, androgens are banned by nearly all major sports organizing bodies. Furthermore, they are listed as Schedule III drugs under the Controlled Substances Act. Modern pharmaceutical chemistry has created several synthetic analogs of the androgens. The goal of creating an analog that retains the muscle-building activity without the adverse effects has not been reached. Testing for the use of new androgen analogs has become a regular part of many major competitive sports, as well at the Olympics.

Erythropoietin is another hormone that is abused by athletes who are attempting to gain a competitive edge. This glycoprotein hormone is normally made by the peritubular cells of the kidney nephrons in response to anoxia or anemia. The target cells of erythropoietin are the hematopoietic cells in the bone marrow that increase the rate of erythrocyte formation in response to erythropoietin. Two recombinant forms of erythropoietin are in use. Epoetin alfa is the normal protein portion of erythropoietin, whereas darbepoetin alfa is a long-acting analog of erythropoietin. Both are used to treat anemia from a variety of causes, and lead to an increase in the patient's hematocrit. In anemic patients, hypertension is the most common adverse effect of both forms.

Abuse of erythropoietin is motivated by the belief that increasing the hematocrit will increase the oxygen-carrying capacity of blood, and, thereby, increase endurance in aerobic activities. The most common sports where this is seen are competitive cycling (most infamously in the Tour de France and other Grand Tour events) and long-distance running and skiing. The effect of increased hematocrit on oxygen transport has been demonstrated in controlled studies [26], but there is still some question of whether this would increase the performance of world-class athletes [27]. Although restoring hematocrit to normal values for anemic patients has few adverse consequences (chiefly hypertension), increasing hematocrit above normal levels carries a significant risk for heart failure, embolism (peripheral and pulmonary), and other thrombosis-related events. The viscosity of blood is increased significantly when the hematocrit increases to above about 50%. This puts significant stress on the heart, an effect that is believed to increase during athletic competition when sweating may lead to a decrease in fluid volume within the body, which increases blood viscosity further. Anecdotally, erythropoietin was implicated in the deaths of 18 cyclists in the 1990s [26], although the drug's use was not proven definitively. For these reasons, erythropoietin use is banned by major sports governing bodies. A test for the use of recombinant erythropoietin relies on the different glycosylation pattern of the recombinant protein, which is manufactured using bacteria to express the cloned gene.

Future trends and summary

Historically, the use of hormones as pharmacotherapeutic agents has followed a consistent pathway. Initially, a native hormone, whether from human or animal tissues, is used. Although these hormones have meant the difference between health and sickness for patients, they often carried a risk for contamination that could lead to other diseases. For example, several cases of iatrogenic Creutzfeldt-Jakob disease have been associated with treatment with hGH [28]. The use of native hormone is followed by synthetic hormones, which carry a much lower risk for causing additional disease. Before the 1980s, synthetic hormones were limited to those that could be synthesized chemically, mainly steroid and simple peptide hormones. The advent of genetic engineering technology allowed the production of large peptide hormones, beginning with insulin. After synthetic hormones were derived, analogs with alterations that were intended to increase the efficacy, duration of effect, or other desirable properties are introduced. These may be a chemically modified version of the native hormone or peptide hormones with altered protein sequences. Most recently, the use of novel chemical techniques has entered the field of drug design. Combinatorial chemistry, in which tens of thousands of chemical variants are tested simultaneously, and computer-aided structural analysis of hormones and their receptors have led to the development of new molecules that act as hormone agonists or antagonists, although the new molecules may bear little relation to the native hormone. At the same time, our understanding of hormones and related chemical messengers in various pathologic conditions continues to grow, and highlight novel targets for new pharmacotherapeutic agents.

The other major change underway is in the modes of administration. Until recently, the rule of thumb was simple. Peptide hormones had to be injected, whereas steroid hormones could be injected, taken orally, applied topically, or inhaled. Several new technologies are under development to increase the available modes. The FDA has approved an inhaled form of insulin for the treatment of diabetes. Other inhalation modes are being explored, as well as the use of molecular delivery systems (eg, liposomes that are able to carry water-soluble molecules across cell membranes). Likewise, the conjugation of drugs to targeting molecules, mainly being developed for cancer therapeutics, could see applications in the targeting of hormones to particular cells or tissues.

In summary, the use of hormones and hormone-related molecules as pharmacotherapeutic agents is an important subset of pharmacology. It makes use of our ever-growing understanding of the homeostatic mechanisms of the human body, and promises to continue to supply new medications.

Acknowledgments

We thank June Hart Romeo for allowing us the opportunity to prepare this review. We also thank Michelle Clapham for her critical reading of this manuscript.

References

[1] Lehne RA. Pharmacology for nursing care. 5th ed. St. Louis (MO): W.B. Saunders; 2004.

[2] Wikipedia. Available at: http://en.wikipedia.org. Accessed May 7, 2006.

[3] Thomas CL, editor. Taber's cyclopedic medical dictionary. 17th ed. Philadelphia: F.A. Davis Company; 1993.

[4] Vincent JL, Zhang H, Szabo C, Preiser JC. Effects of nitric oxide in septic shock. Am J Respir Crit Care Med 2000;161:1781–5.

[5] Kenakin T. Predicting therapeutic value in the lead optimization phase of drug discovery. Nat Rev Drug Discov 2003;2:429–38.

[6] Howlett AC. A short guide to the nomenclature of seven-transmembrane spanning receptors for lipid mediators. Life Sci 2005;77:1522–30.

[7] FDA approves first ever inhaled insulin combination product for treatment of diabetes. Available at: http://www.fda.gov/bbs/topics/news/2006/NEW01304.html. Accessed May 7, 2006.

[8] Wikipedia. Growth hormone treatment. Available at: http://en.wikipedia.org/wiki/Growth_hormone_treatment. Accessed May 7, 2006.

[9] Allen DB, Fost N. hGH for short stature: ethical issues raised by expanded access. J Pediatr 2004;144:648–52.

[10] Sandberg DE, Colsman M. Growth hormone treatment of short stature: status of the quality of life rationale. Horm Res 2005;63:275–83.

[11] Bunevicius R, Kazanavicius G, Zalinkevicius R, et al. Effects of thyroxine as compared with thyroxine plus triiodothyronine in patients with hypothyroidism. N Engl J Med 1999;340:424–9.

[12] Women's Health Initiative home page. Available at: http://www.nhlbi.nih.gov/whi/index.html. Accessed May 13, 2006.

[13] Estrogen and estrogen with progestin therapies for postmenopausal women. Available at: http://www.fda.gov/cder/drug/infopage/estrogens_progestins/default.htm. Accessed May 16, 2006.

[14] Chlebowski RT, Hendrix SL, Langer RD, et al. Influence of estrogen plus progestin on breast cancer and mammography in healthy postmenopausal women: the Women's Health Initiative Randomized Trial. JAMA 2003;289:3243–53.

[15] Stefanick ML, Anderson GL, Margolis KL, et al. Effects of conjugated equine estrogens on breast cancer and mammography screening in postmenopausal women with hysterectomy. JAMA 2006;295:1647–57.

[16] Women's Health Initiative Fact Sheet. Available at: http://www.nhlbi.nih.gov/whi/factsht.htm. Accessed May 15, 2006.

[17] Wenzel V, Krismer AC, Arntz HR, et al. A comparison of vasopressin and epinephrine for out-of-hospital cardiopulmonary resuscitation. N Engl J Med 2004;350:105–13.

[18] Rudman D, Feller AG, Nagraj HS, et al. Effects of human growth hormone in men over 60 years old. N Engl J Med 1990;323:1–6.

[19] Vance ML. Can growth hormone prevent aging? N Engl J Med 2003;348:779–80.

[20] Perls TT, Reisman NR, Olshansky SJ. Provision or distribution of growth hormone for "antiaging": clinical and legal issues. JAMA 2005;294:2086–90.

[21] Coursin DB, Wood KE. Corticosteroid supplementation for adrenal insufficiency. JAMA 2002;287:236–40.

[22] Almawi WY, bou Jaoude MM, Li XC. Transcriptional and post-transcriptional mechanisms of glucocorticoid antiproliferative effects. Hematol Oncol 2002;20:17–32.

[23] Antony PA, Restifo NP. CD4$^+$CD25$^+$ T regulatory cells, immunotherapy of cancer, and interleukin-2. J Immunother 2005;28:120–8.

[24] King DS, Sharp RL, Vukovich MD, et al. Effect of oral androstenedione on serum testosterone and adaptations to resistance training in young men: a randomized controlled trial. JAMA 1999;281:2020–8.

[25] Bhasin S, Storer TW, Berman N, et al. The effects of supraphysiologic doses of testosterone on muscle size and strength in normal men. N Engl J Med 1996;335:1–7.

[26] Jelkmann W. Use of recombinant human erythropoietin as an antianemic and performance enhancing drug. Curr Pharm Biotechnol 2000;1:11–31.

[27] Spivak JL. Erythropoietin use and abuse. In: Roach RR, Wagner PD, Hackett PH, editors. Hypoxia: from genes to the bedside. New York: Kluwer Academic/Plenum Publishers; 2001. p. 207–24.

[28] Cordery RJ, Hall M, Cipolotti L, et al. Early cognitive decline in Creutzfeldt-Jakob disease associated with human growth hormone treatment. J Neurol Neurosurg Psychiatry 2003;74: 1412–6.

ELSEVIER
SAUNDERS

Nurs Clin N Am 42 (2007) 19–27

NURSING
CLINICS
OF NORTH AMERICA

Hypovitaminosis D and Morbid Obesity

Juan Ybarra, MD, PhD, FACE[a],*,
Joan Sánchez-Hernández, MD, PhD[a,b],
Antonio Pérez, MD, PhD[b]

[a]*Servicio de Endocrinología y Nutrición, Hospital de Sant Pau,*
Mas Casanovas 90, Barcelona 08041, Spain
[b]*Departamento de Medicina, Universitat Autònoma de Barcelona, Barcelona, Spain*

Obesity is by far the most prevalent metabolic disease worldwide. Hence, the World Health Organization calls it an epidemic, given its prevalence, incidence, and socio-sanitary burden. These epidemiologic considerations, along with the improvements in safety and efficiency of bariatric surgery, the increasing patient demand, and health care providers' sensibility, explain why an increasing number of premorbid and morbidly obese patients undergo this type of surgical procedure. Bariatric surgery permits weight loss through restrictive techniques (vertical banded gastroplasty), malabsorptive techniques (biliopancreatic bypass), or mixed procedures (gastric bypass). Generally, the greatest weight loss is achieved using malabsorptive or mixed procedures [1]. Nevertheless, these surgical modalities carry side effects and complications of which we need to be aware.

Vitamin D deficiency is one of the alterations that is related most frequently to malabsorptive bariatric techniques [2]. This is understandable because vitamin D is absorbed passively [3], although it also is dependent upon biliary salts and calcium metabolism, which facilitate its absorption.

Vitamin D insufficiency in the adult results in osteomalacia, which is characterized by a defect in bone mineralization with a simultaneous increase in osteoid formation. Its clinical expression includes bony pains, muscular weakness secondary to proximal myotonia, pseudofractures, and, in late stages, gait disturbances similar to those encountered in fibromyalgia or polymyalgia rheumatica [4].

Early diagnosis is paramount because chronic vitamin D deficits are associated with nonreversible bony structural modifications. Hence, laboratory findings, including elevated serum alkaline phosphatase levels, coupled

---

* Corresponding author.
E-mail address: juanybarra@hotmail.com (J. Ybarra).

0029-6465/07/$ - see front matter © 2007 Elsevier Inc. All rights reserved.
doi:10.1016/j.cnur.2006.12.001
nursing.theclinics.com

with diminished circulating 25-OH-vitamin D and diminished urinary calcium excretion, alert us to a stage precluding osteomalacia, which is reversible with calcium and vitamin D supplementation [5].

Vitamin D and parathyroid hormone physiopathology

Calcium is absorbed primarily at the duodenum and jejunum. Its absorption capacity is determined by the bioavailability and total amount of dietary calcium. The main sources of dietary calcium are cheese and dairy products, although vegetables also provide us with calcium; nevertheless, its bioavailability is hampered by the binding of dietary fiber, phytic acid (inositol phosphate), and oxalates [3]. Most dietary calcium is absorbed by vitamin D–mediated transcellular diffusion, and under normal circumstances, approximately 30% of dietary calcium is absorbed.

The most frequent causes of impaired calcium absorption include poor calcium intake, vitamin D deficiency, and lack of intestinal response to vitamin D (eg, glucocorticoid excess, thyroid hormone excess, malabsorption syndromes).

Vitamin D synthesis starts with ultraviolet radiation on skin 7-dehydrocholesterol, which is converted to previtamin D3; this, in turn, is transformed to vitamin D3 (cholecalciferol). This vitamin D3 and a certain amount of the dietary vitamin D3 undergo 25-hydroxylation at the liver to yield 25-(OH)D3 or calcidiol, which is the main circulating form of vitamin D. Calcidiol undergoes renal 1-α-hydroxylation to yield 1α,25-dihydroxyvitamin D (calcitriol), which is the more active form of vitamin D. Parathyroid hormone (PTH), hypocalcemia (through PTH stimulation), and hyperphosphatemia enhance calcitriol production. Furthermore, liver diseases may impair 25-hydroxylation, and renal diseases may suppress 1-α-hydroxylation. Other hormones, such as prolactin, growth hormone, and sex steroids, also modulate calcitriol production.

24-25(OH)^{2}D3, whose physiologic role is not known, is another kidney end product of calcidiol.

Calcitriol exerts its actions in the same fabrics as does PTH, but its subcellular sites and mechanism of action are different. Unlike PTH, which interacts with a recipient in the extracellular membrane, calcitriol joins an intracellular recipient, and the complex is fixed to specific sites in the chromatin [6,7]. At these particular sites, calcitriol acts as a steroid hormone.

In the gut, calcitriol stimulates the synthesis of a calcium-binding protein and stimulates calcium and phosphorus absorption, although a clear interplay among the latter and its effects has not been elucidated [8,9].

When calcium and phosphorus serum concentrations increase, calcitriol promotes their deposition in bone hydroxylapatite and, paradoxically, removes calcium from the formed bone. Additionally, calcitriol inhibits the synthesis of prepro-PTH and may well be a physiologic regulator of PTH synthesis and secretion.

Calcitriol receptors are ubiquitous in tissues other than bone, kidney, and intestine, including parathyroid and mammary glands, pancreatic islets, fibroblasts, and other tissues not belonging to the classic calcitriol target tissues [10].

Calcidiol has a longer plasma half-life than calcitriol and more stable concentrations, which make its measurements the most valuable for assessing vitamin D metabolism and status in daily clinical practice. The accepted normal values range from 38 to 125 nmol/L. Low calcidiol levels are encountered frequently during pregnancy, hyperthyroidism, anticonvulsant treatment, and other states. Increased calcidiol levels are seen rarely and confirm vitamin D intoxication.

There is much less experience with measuring calcitriol levels. Its regulation is different from that of calcidiol. Moreover, its normal range is reduced ($\times 1000$) and ranges from 43 to 150 pmol/L. It is influenced by age (lower levels with advanced age), season (lower levels in winter), serum calcium levels, and other less clearly established factors. PTH augments calcitriol concentration whenever kidney function is intact. The latter makes calcitriol useful in the differential diagnosis of hypercalcemia [11].

Vitamin D deficiency may be secondary to insufficient dietary intake or diminished absorption due to hepatobiliary or intestinal malabsorption. Additionally, it may be secondary to drug-induced alterations of vitamin D metabolism (ie, phenobarbital, diphenylhydantoin, rifampicin) or sunlight underexposure. The latter is an important acquired form of vitamin D deficiency in Nordic countries and in individuals whose skin rarely is exposed to sunlight.

Type I vitamin D–dependent rickets is a recessive autosomal disease in which there is a deficit of 1-α-hydroxylase enzyme (needed to convert calcidiol into calcitriol). Conversely, in type II vitamin D–dependent rickets, target organs cannot respond to 1α,25-dihydroxy-vitamin D. The most frequent causes of vitamin D deficiency include:

Inadequate dietary intake
Sunlight underexposure
Renal disease
Hepatobiliary disease
Pancreatic disease
Intestinal malabsorption
Cancer
Drugs
Type I and II vitamin D–dependent rickets

Secondary hyperparathyroidism is the result of the parathyroid glands adaptation to chronic renal insufficiency. This condition invariably leads to diminished calcitriol production, diminished calcitriol-mediated calcium absorption and hypocalcemia, and, finally, hyperphosphatemia due to renal mass loss. Hypocalcemia and hyperphosphatemia stimulate parathyroid function. Other causes of secondary hyperparathyroidism include renal and bone resistance to PTH and gastrointestinal diseases that induce calcium and vitamin D malabsorption [2,12]. Because PTH hypersecretion is an adaptative, rather than autonomous, phenomenon, it rarely causes hypercalcemia [2]. On the contrary, we assume there is parathyroid compensation whenever serum calcium is diminished or within abnormally normal serum levels. The radiologic finding of osteitis fibrosa cystica offers additional information in this particular clinical setting [13].

PTH measurement usually provides confirmatory results of hyperparathyroidism, although its interpretation may be confusing in some patients because of quantitative and qualitative differences in the laboratory techniques used (ie, methods measuring carboxy-terminal PTH fragments versus amino-terminal PTH fragments).

Definition of hypovitaminosis D

Generally, serum calcidiol levels are measured using radioimmune analysis with a reference range of 25 to 150 nmol/L. Vitamin D deficiency corresponds to serum calcidiol levels less than 25 nmol/L. In this situation, there is accompanying secondary hyperparathyroidism and clinical osteopathy. Vitamin D insufficiency corresponds to serum calcidiol levels in the range of 25 to 50 nmol/L, with accompanying secondary hyperparathyroidism but without clinical osteopathy. If vitamin D insufficiency is sustained for prolonged periods, it may result in clinical osteopathy. Serum calcidiol levels greater than 50 nmol/L are considered normal (Box 1) [13]; however, there is some controversy about levels between 50 to 100 nmol/L because hypovitaminosis D has been described within this range (Table 1) [14]. Furthermore, other vitamin D experts agree on sufficient vitamin D levels with serum calcidiol concentrations greater than 31 ng/mL [15,16], based on epidemiologic studies in which circulating PTH levels (>36 pg/mL) appeared only in subjects with calcidiol levels less than the 31 ng/mL cutoff [17].

Box 1. Calcidiol ranges stratification

Deficient <25 nmol/L
Insufficient 25–50 nmol/L
Normal >50 nmol/L

Data from Lips P. Vitamin D deficiency and secondary hyperparathyroidism in the elderly: consequences for bone loss and fractures and therapeutic implications. Endocr Rev 2001;22;477–501.

Table 1
Calcidiol ranges stratification

Calcidiol	Deficient	Insufficient	Hypovitaminosis D	Desirable
nmol/L	<25	25–50	50–100	>100
ng/mL	<10	10–20	20–40	>40

Data from MacKenna M, Freaney R. Secondary hyperparathyroidism in the elderly: means to defining hypovitaminosis D. Osteoporos Int 1998;8(Suppl):S3–6.

Obesity and hypovitaminosis D

The available data on vitamin D levels in morbidly obese patients are scarce and flawed; in most instances, vitamin D deficiency was blamed on previous bariatric surgery, without consideration that the deficit may have preceded surgery [1]. Hence, vitamin D deficiency and secondary hyperparathyroidism in association with morbid obesity have been described in patients who did and did not undergo bariatric surgery [18–22]. Moreover, recent studies suggest that surgery does not significantly account for this deficiency [23,24].

Some observational studies reported inversely proportional relationships between calcium, vitamin D, and body mass index [25–27]. Moreover, more recently, hypovitaminosis D has been linked with obesity-associated syndromes, such as syndrome X, high blood pressure, and type 2 diabetes mellitus, among others [16,28–30]. Conversely, other studies suggested that diets rich in vitamin D and calcium can potentiate postprandial thermogenesis and lipid oxidation [31].

There is not a single unifying hypothesis to explain why obese patients tend to display vitamin D deficiency. Conversely, several pathophysiologic mechanisms are well described in morbidly obese patients who have not undergone bariatric surgery that partially explain vitamin D deficits, including the negative feedback on hepatic 25-OH-vitamin D synthesis [18], sunlight underexposure [20], and diminished bioavailability of vitamin D that is due to enhanced uptake by adipose tissue [15].

Bariatric surgery and hypovitaminosis D

By far, the long-term outcomes of bariatric surgery have exceeded those of any other therapeutic option; the individual is provided with structural modifications that lie well beyond one's will power and include restricted food intake or malabsorption of the latter.

The main advantage of restrictive procedures is that a reduced amount of well-digested food follows its physiologic pathway, and, thus, has virtually no nutritional and vitamin deficits. Mixed procedures, combining restriction and malabsorption, slow the mixture of food intake with bile and pancreatic juice. The result is early satiety combined with a sense of satisfaction that reduces hunger.

Pure malabsorptive techniques allow a greater weight reduction, despite larger amounts of food intake. The associated risks include potential protein and vitamin deficits, anemia, and bone disease.

Early postoperative complications after Roux-en-Y gastric bypass—the most frequently performed mixed bariatric surgery technique [1]—include multiple vitamin and micronutrient deficiencies (ie, iron, vitamin B12, folic acid, calcium, and vitamin D). Late complications include, among others, 73% of metabolic bone disease [32].

According to previous reports, the pathogenesis of metabolic bone disease would be secondary to vitamin D and calcium malabsorption [13]; nevertheless, data extrapolated from bariatric studies using restrictive or mixed techniques do not support the previous hypothesis, and vitamin D levels are unchanged postoperatively. Moreover, obese patients' bone mineral densities are higher compared with controls, suggesting that there is an adaptation of the skeleton to increased weight bearing [33,34].

Despite this controversy, the prevalence of vitamin D deficiency is high in patients who have undergone bariatric surgery, particularly if the procedure implied malabsorption. Several longitudinal studies reported calcium and vitamin D depletion in patients who had undergone bariatric surgery at mid- and long-term follow-up. The incidence of those deficits was maximal with older malabsorptive techniques (ie, jejunoileal bypass) and on the degree of malabsorption achieved [32,35–40]. The authors' group noted that vitamin D deficiency was present, in most cases, before surgery [23]. The first cross-sectional results allowed the authors to suggest that bariatric surgery was unlikely to alter the previous deficits significantly. Hence, they studied 180 patients who had and had not undergone bariatric surgery. The patients were classified into three categories (normal, insufficient, and deficient) according to serum calcidiol levels. Hypovitaminosis D was present in 79.8% of patients (46.8% insufficient, 33% deficient). There were no significant differences between the groups that did and did not undergo surgery.

Table 2
Calcidiol status in three different categories (normal, insufficient and deficient) depending on circulation serum levels in the operative versus the nonoperative group

	Calcidiol status			
	Normal (>50 nmol/L)	Insufficient (25–50 nmol/L)	Deficient (<25 nmol/L)	Total
Surgery	22.7%	34.1%	43.2%	100%
Nosurgery	18.8%	53.8%	27.5%	100%
Total	20.2%	46.8%	33.1%	100%

Data from Ybarra J, Sánchez-Hernández J, Gich I, et al. Unchanged hypovitaminosis D and secondary hyperparathyroidism in morbid obesity after bariatric surgery. Obes Surg 2005; 15:330–5.

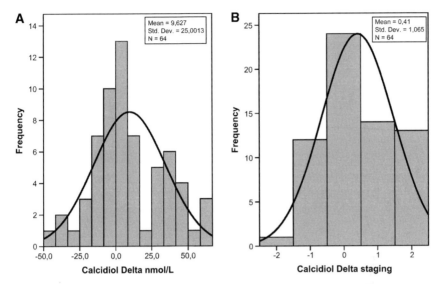

Fig. 1. Differences in calcidiol levels (*A*) and stages (*B*) before and after bariatric surgery. (*From* Sánchez-Hernández J, Ybarra J, Gich I, et al. Effects of bariatric surgery on vitamin D status and secondary hyperparathyroidism: a prospective study. Obes Surg 2005;15:1389–95; with kind permission of Springer Science and Business Media.)

Thus, 77.3% of patients in the surgical group presented with hypovitaminosis D (34.1% insufficient, 43.2% deficient), whereas 81.2% of patients in the nonsurgical group presented with hypovitaminosis D (53.8% insufficient, 27.4% deficient). Conversely, only 20.2% of the studied population had normal calcidiol levels, and there were not a significant difference between the groups (surgical = 22.7% versus nonsurgical = 18.8%) (Table 2) [23].

The authors' second study evaluated changes in calcidiol levels longitudinally from baseline (before bariatric surgery) to 36 months of follow-up in morbidly obese patients who did not receive calcium or vitamin D supplementation. Almost 80% of the cohort had stable or increased calcidiol levels, whereas only 20% had decreased calcidiol levels (Fig. 1) [24].

Taken together, the results of the authors' two studies [23,24] suggest that hypovitaminosis D in morbidly obese patients precedes bariatric surgery; thus, surgery, by itself, is unlikely to be exclusively responsible for hypovitaminosis D. Furthermore, in almost every morbidly obese patient who has postoperative hypovitaminosis D, the deficit and its clinical symptoms are entirely reversible upon calcium and vitamin D supplementation [4,33,40].

Summary

Despite the belief that hypovitaminosis D is one of the most frequent complications of bariatric surgery, the available data strongly suggest that in most patients, the deficit precedes surgery. Thus, taking into account the elevated prevalence of hypovitaminosis D, the associated morbidity, and the availability of efficient treatments to reverse the biochemical and clinical scenario, it seems reasonable to recommend routine monitoring of serum levels of calcium, phosphorus, and vitamin D in morbidly obese patients and to supplement with calcium and vitamin D whenever necessary.

References

[1] Chapin BL, LeMar HJ, Knodel DH, et al. Secondary hyperparathyroidism following biliopancreatic diversion. Arch Surg 1996;113:1048–52.

[2] Guangiroli M. Cirugías malabsortivas. Argentina: Facultad Favoloro Argentina Press; 2004.

[3] Marsh M, Ryley S. Enfermedades gastrointestinales y hepáticas. Panamericana 1998;cap 87:1577–608.

[4] Goldner W, O'Dorisio T, Dillon J, et al. Severe metabolic bone disease as a long-term complication of obesity surgery. Obes Surg 2002;12:685–92.

[5] Basha B, Rao S, Han Z, et al. Osteomalacia due to vitamin D depletion: a neglected consequence of intestinal malabsorption. Am J Med 2000;108:296–300.

[6] Kawashima H, Kurokawa K. Metabolism and sites of action of vitamin D in the kidney. Kidney Int 1986;29:98–107.

[7] Kumar R. The metabolism and mechanism of action of 1,25-dihydroxyvitamin D3. Kidney Int 1986;30:793–803.

[8] Reichel H, Koeffler HP, Norman AW. The role of the vitamin D endocrine system in health and disease. N Engl J Med 1989;320:980.

[9] Norman AW, Roth J, Orci L. The vitamin D endocrine system: steroid metabolism, hormone receptors, and biological response (calcium binding proteins). Endocr Rev 1982;3:331.

[10] DeLuca HF, Krisinger J, Darwish H. The vitamin D system: 1990. Kidney Int 1990; 38(Suppl 29):S2–8.

[11] MacIntyre I, Alevizaki M, Bevis PJR, et al. Calcitonin and the peptides from the calcitonine gene. Clin Orthop 1987;217:45–55.

[12] Delmez JA, Slatopolsky E. Recent advances in the pathogenesis and therapy of uremic secondary hyperparathyroidism. J Clin Endocrinol Metab 1991;72:735.

[13] Lips P. Vitamin D deficiency and secondary hyperparathyroidism in the elderly: consequences for bone loss and fractures and therapeutic implications. Endocr Rev 2001;22: 477–501.

[14] MacKenna M, Freaney R. Secondary hyperparathyroidism in the elderly: means to defining hypovitaminosis D. Osteoporos Int 1998;8(Suppl):S3–6.

[15] Wortsman J, Matsuoka LY, Chen TC, et al. Decreased bioavailability of vitamin D in obesity. Am J Nutr 2000;72:690–3.

[16] Holick MF. Vitamin D: the underappreciated D-lightful hormone that is important for skeletal and cellular health. Curr Opin Endocrinol Diabetes 2002;9:87–98.

[17] Chapuy MC, Shott AM, Garnero P, et al. Healthy elderly French women living at home have secondary hyperparathyroidism and high bone turnover in winter. Endocrinol Metab 1996; 81:1129–33.

[18] Bell NH, Epstein S, Greene A, et al. Evidence for alteration of the vitamin D-endocrine system in obese subjects. J Clin Invest 1985;76:370–3.

[19] Liel Y, Ulmer E, Shary J, et al. Low circulating vitamin D in obesity. Calcif Tissue Int 1988; 43:199–201.

[20] Compston JE, Vedi S, Ledger JE, et al. Vitamin D status and bone histomorphometry in gross obesity. Am J Nutr 1981;34:2359–63.

[21] Hey HE, Stockholm KH, Lun BJ, et al. Vitamin D deficiency in obese patients and changes in circulating vitamin D metabolism following jejunoileal bypass. Int J Obes 1982;6:473–9.

[22] Hyldstrup L, Andersen T, McNair P, et al. Bone metabolism in obesity: changes related to severe overweight and dietary weight reduction. Acta Endocrinol (Copenh) 1993;129:393–8.

[23] Ybarra J, Sánchez-Hernández J, Gich I, et al. Unchanged hypovitaminosis D and secondary hyperparathyroidism in morbid obesity after bariatric surgery. Obes Surg 2005;15:330–5.

[24] Sánchez-Hernández J, Ybarra J, Gich I, et al. Effects of bariatric surgery on vitamin D status and secondary hyperparathyroidism: a prospective study. Obes Surg 2005;15:1389–95.

[25] Buffington C, Walker B, Cowan GS Jr, et al. Vitamin D deficiency in the morbidly obese. Obes Surg 1993;3(4):421–4.

[26] Heaney RP, Davies KM, Barger-Lux MJ. Calcium and weight: clinical studies. J Am Coll Nutr 2002;21(2):152S–5S.

[27] Kamycheva E, Sundsfjord J, Jorde R. Serum parathyroid hormone level is associated with body mass index. The 5th Tromso Study. Eur J Endocrinol 2004;151(2):167–72.

[28] Liu S, Song Y, Ford ES, et al. Dietary calcium, vitamin D, and the prevalence of metabolic syndrome in middle-aged and older US women. Diabetes Care 2005;28:2926–32.

[29] Holick MF. Calcium and vitamin D. Diagnostics and therapeutics. Clin Lab Med 2000; 20:569–90.

[30] De Prisco C, Levine SN. Metabolic bone disease after gastric bypass surgery for obesity. Am J Med 2005;118:51–7.

[31] Ping-Delfos WC, Soares MJ, Cummings NK. Acute suppression of spontaneous food intake following dairy calcium and vitamin D. Asia Pac J Clin Nutr 2004;13(Suppl):S82.

[32] Compston JE, Vedi S, Gianetta E, et al. Bone histomorphometry and vitamin D status after biliopancreatic bypass for obesity. Gastroenterology 1984;87(2):350–6.

[33] Scopinaro N, Adami GF, Marinari G, et al. Biliopancreatic diversion: two decades of experience. In: Update: surgery for the morbidly obese patient. 2000. p. 227–58.

[34] Guney E, Kisakol G, Yilmaz C, et al. Effect of weight loss on bone metabolism: comparison of vertical banded gastroplasty and medical intervention. Obes Surg 2003;13:383–8.

[35] Teitelbaum SL, Halverson JD, Bates M, et al. Abnormalities of circulating 25-OH vitamin D after jejuno-ileal bypass for obesity. Ann Intern Med 1977;86:289–93.

[36] Compston JE, Laker MF, Woodhead JS, et al. Bone disease after jejunoileal bypass for obesity. Lancet 1978;2:1–4.

[37] Parfitt AM, Miller JM, Frame B, et al. Metabolic bone disease after intestinal bypass for treatment of obesity. Ann Intern Med 1978;89:193–9.

[38] Hey H, Stokholm KH, Lund BJ, et al. Vitamin D deficiency in obese patients and changes in circulating vitamin D metabolites following jejunoileal bypass. Int J Obes 1982;6:473–9.

[39] Hamoui N, Kim K, Anthone G, et al. The significance of elevated levels of parathyroid hormone in patients with morbid obesity before and after bariatric surgery. Arch Surg 2003;138:891–7.

[40] Newbury L, Dolan K, Hatzifotis M, et al. Calcium and vitamin D depletion and elevated parathyroid hormone following biliopancreatic diversion. Obes Surg 2003;13:893–5.

ELSEVIER
SAUNDERS

NURSING
CLINICS
OF NORTH AMERICA

Nurs Clin N Am 42 (2007) 29–42

A Cascade of Events – Obesity, Metabolic Syndrome, and Type 2 Diabetes Mellitus in Youth

Ruth C. McGillis Bindler, RNC, PhD

Washington State University/Intercollegiate College of Nursing, West 2917
Fort George Wright Drive, Spokane, WA 99224, USA

Increased rates of obesity among youth have emerged in the last 2 to 3 decades in the United States and in developed countries around the world. More recently, these trends have emerged even in very young children, and have become magnified among all child and adolescent age groups. Initially, it was unknown what related health outcomes would arise in youth, although the relationships of obesity in adults to outcomes such as increased cardiovascular disease, type 2 diabetes, orthopedic problems, certain cancers, polycystic ovarian disease, and a myriad of other conditions, had been well documented. It is now known that youth share in at least several of the health outcomes that are related to obesity. This article focuses on two of those outcomes, namely metabolic syndrome and type 2 diabetes mellitus (T2DM).

The growing incidence of obesity and its related health problems can be viewed as a cascade. Imagine a water cascade that pours out of its source, gathering momentum as it tumbles downhill. Springs add to the surging water as it cascades and falls in an unstoppable manner. Obesity is the starting point of a seemingly unstoppable cascade of health events. It surges through a population of youth, gathering momentum from environmental factors, such as decreased physical activity and increased consumption of sugared beverages. It tumbles downward, spiraling into dark areas representative of metabolic syndrome and T2DM. Although seemingly out of control, a cascade can be harnessed. A dam can be built, conduits can displace water from its path, and springs can be diverted elsewhere. Similarly, many types of interventions can be used to interrupt obesity and its health outcomes. Using several strategies likely will be the best approach to stop the cascade

E-mail address: bindler@wsu.edu

of unhealthy events that follow obesity in youth. This article reviews the incidence of, and contributors to, youth obesity, the emergence of metabolic syndrome and type 2 diabetes in relationship with weight, and the prevention, assessment, and intervention approaches that can be applied with youth to interrupt obesity and the cascade of associated conditions.

Obesity in youth

Obesity in youth is defined differently than in adults. Height and weight are measured, and body mass index (BMI) is calculated as a ratio of weight to height (kg/m^2). The resultant number must be placed on a BMI growth grid, consistent with the child's gender and age, to determine the BMI percentile. It is recommended that youth have a BMI between the 5th and 85th percentiles. Youth with BMI between the 85th and 95th percentiles are considered overweight, and those with BMI above the 95th percentile are defined as obese [1]. Some practitioners prefer not to use the term "obesity" with children because of its negative connotations; they use the term "at risk for overweight" for the 85th to 95th percentiles, and the term "overweight" for youth whose BMI is above the 95th percentile [2].

Youth rates of obesity had remained stable in the United States at approximately 4% to 7% for many years, but began a precipitous increase in the 1980s. In the 1988–1994 National Health and Nutrition Examination Surveys (NHANES), 11% of children from 6 to 19 years were identified as having a BMI at or above the 95th percentile; 1999–2002 data revealed that 16% were above that level [3]. Data available for 2003–2004 indicate that 17.1% of youth from 2 to 19 years are above the 95th percentile [4]. This upward trend seems to be continuing, and is mirrored in Canada and other countries worldwide. Even the very youngest children are increasingly affected, with approximately 10% of 2- to 5-year-old children now above the 95th percentile for BMI [5]. In selected samples, the prevalence of excessive BMI is even higher. For example, in a study of 3- to 5-year-olds in Chicago, 24% had BMI that was above the 95th percentile [6]. The trend of excess weight in the very young is especially disturbing, because patterns of obesity tend to persist over time, and because the potential burden of associated health problems is magnified when obesity begins so early in development.

Childhood obesity is now identified as an epidemic. The increase in incidence of excessive weight in children is troubling because it is accompanied by an interruption in a state of well-being and increased risks for numerous health problems. Health problems include social and emotional sequelae, such as depression, low self-esteem, negative body image, and discrimination; cardiovascular complications, such as hypertension, left ventricular hypertrophy, and atherosclerosis; metabolic conditions, such as insulin resistance, metabolic syndrome, and dyslipidemia; pulmonary problems, such as asthma, obstructive sleep apnea, and obesity hypoventilation syndrome; musculoskeletal problems, such as fractures, Blount disease, and slipped capital femoral epiphysis; and other conditions, such as gastroesophageal reflux, cholelithiasis, hepatitic steatosis, polycystic ovarian syndrome, and pseudotumor cerebri [2,5,7].

Research has focused on identifying the incidence of obesity among youth of various ages, racial and ethnic groups, and socioeconomic and geographic backgrounds. Although obesity has increased across all age, race, and ethnic groups, children from families with low incomes, and those from minority racial/ethnic groups have higher rates of obesity [5,7]. The contributors to the epidemic of obesity, such as increased caloric intake, reliance on fast foods, decreases in physical activity, and environmental design (eg, neighborhoods without sidewalks and absence of essential services within walking distance), have been examined. The role of genetics as a risk factor also is being explored. More recently, a focus on prevention and intervention programs has emerged as health practitioners seek to reverse, or at least staunch, the obesity epidemic.

Metabolic syndrome

Metabolic syndrome was identified first in adults by Reaven [8], who defined a series of events that tended to cluster in individuals; the coexistence of these symptoms was variously labeled as syndrome X, insulin resistance syndrome, or dysmetabolic syndrome. In the United States, the Adult Treatment Panel III of the National Cholesterol Education Program recommends that the syndrome be diagnosed in adults when three of five criteria are present: hypertriglyceridemia, low high-density lipoprotein cholesterol (HDL-C), high fasting blood glucose, hypertension, and high waist circumference. The World Health Organization and the International Diabetes Federation use slightly different criteria [9]. No clear set of criteria and cutoffs has been applied to youth, but practitioners have adapted the adult criteria in several ways for application to younger age groups [10,11].

Regardless of the specific criteria that are applied to diagnose metabolic syndrome in youth, its incidence is clearly increasing. An investigation that analyzed the same metabolic syndrome criteria using NHANES data from 1988–1992 and from 1999–2000 found that the prevalence of metabolic syndrome had increased from 4.2% to 6.4% in that short span [12]. It also is notable that the prevalence of metabolic syndrome is 28.7% in adolescents in at least the 95th percentile for BMI, compared with 6.1% for those in the 85th to 95th percentiles, and 0.1% for those less in than the 85th percentile [13]. The most common criterion identified for the syndrome in overweight youth was abdominal obesity, followed by hypertriglyceridemia, low HDL-C, and high blood pressure (BP). Impaired fasting glucose was the least common criterion among youth [13]. Another study of 588 obese white children found that 23.3% had metabolic syndrome [14]. The metabolic syndrome is associated clearly with obesity, and indeed, is rarely seen without the manifestation of excess weight.

Insulin resistance is the cardinal metabolic factor that underlies the body changes that can be observed and measured easily. Insulin activity represents a complex system, depending on enzymes, feedback loops, and other factors. Insulin is secreted by the β cells of the pancreas. It binds to receptors on the surfaces of cells where it assists in relocating transporter proteins from intracellular to plasma membranes, thereby facilitating transfer of glucose across the cell membranes. Although some tissues can transport glucose without the presence of insulin, many, such as adipose tissue, skeletal muscle, and heart muscle, are dependent on insulin for glucose transfer. Insulin also affects intracellular glucose metabolism and promotes glycogen synthesis. Obesity seems to decrease the number of insulin receptors on the cell surface, a condition known as insulin resistance. The pancreas attempts to compensate for this condition by secreting more insulin, which leads to hyperinsulinemia. Eventually, the pancreas is unable to meet the high need for insulin production and fails; this leads to diabetes. The level of insulin resistance and the timing of the failure are influenced by genetics [15,16]. In one study of nearly 500 youth, those of normal weight had an average serum insulin level of 10.3 μU/mL, those overweight had a mean level of 14.6 μU/mL, and those severely obese had a level of 38.6 μU/mL [17].

Although the state of insulin resistance is worsening, the body's maintenance of a steady state of glucose falters. Impaired glucose tolerance (IGT) reflects the inability to maintain glucose within normal levels. Clinicians administer postprandial plasma glucose or oral glucose tolerance tests for diagnosis of IGT [18]. A 2-hour postprandial blood glucose of 140 to 199 mg/dL is indicative of IGT [19], a state referred to as prediabetes.

The conditions of insulin resistance and hyperinsulinemia contribute directly to the metabolic syndrome criteria of hypertriglyceridemia and low HDL-C, as well as high BP. High insulin levels facilitate free fatty acid release from adipose tissue and influence the liver to increase triglyceride manufacture. Hyperinsulinemia also increases renal sodium retention, decreases uric acid clearance, and results in hypertension [20]. Elevated insulin levels also contribute to another biologic marker that is not one of the major criteria for metabolic syndrome but is recognized as a clear signal that elevated insulin is present. Acanthosis nigricans (AN) is a darkening of the skin in areas of skinfolds, such as axilla, neck, groin, and between fingers. In a study of adolescents, 34% of those who had AN also had elevated serum insulin levels; when an elevated BMI also was present, almost 50% had elevated insulin [21]. Additional factors, such as albumin excretion, plasma uric acid, fibrinogen, plasminogen activator inhibitor type 1, C-reactive protein, interleukin 6, adiponectin, and very-low-density lipoprotein cholesterol, are being investigated as markers of metabolic syndrome.

Thus, one can view the state of being overweight and that of insulin resistance as coexisting and contributing to each other. They lead to hyperinsulinemia, a condition that can be identified by serum insulin levels and sometimes by AN. The condition also influences the development of increased triglycerides, low HDL-C, and hypertension, primary markers of the syndrome. Although serum glucose elevations may be seen in adults, they are slow to develop, and, therefore, are not a good criterion for the syndrome in youth.

Type 2 diabetes mellitus

T2DM is a disease that occurs when insulin resistance at the cellular level cannot be overcome by production of increased amounts of insulin by the β cells of the pancreas. The pancreas finally fails to secrete adequate insulin; initially postprandial, and, ultimately, fasting hyperglycemia, become evident [22].

Thereby, the diagnosis of T2DM signals a crashing of the cascade that began with obesity and metabolic syndrome. Even if the present obesity rates do not continue to escalate, 30% of the boys and 40% of the girls who were born in 2000 are expected to be diagnosed with diabetes in their lifetime [23]. If obesity continues to escalate, the incidence could be even greater. Among at-risk ethnic groups, such as Native Americans, African Americans, Hispanics, and Asian/Pacific Islanders, the incidence is significantly greater [24–26].

Formerly, T2DM was called "adult-onset diabetes," indicating that it was nearly undiagnosed in children and adolescents; however, that situation has changed. T2DM has been identified in children throughout the world, and data suggest that from 8% to 45% of new cases of diabetes in children are due to T2DM. Accurate population-based data are not available on incidence, but estimates range from about 4 to 7 per 1000 in United States adolescents [7,27,28]. In all samples studied, the incidence is increasing at a rapid rate [22]. For example, during the 1990s, the number of Native American and Alaska Native children who were diagnosed with diabetes increased 73%; even when considering all ethnic groups, there was a 60% increase in diabetes rates among adolescent girls and an 81% increase among adolescent boys [29]. Great variation can occur in different parts of the country and for different tribes of native peoples. The incidence of T2DM ranges from 2.3 per 1000 for Canadian First Nation people in Manitoba to 4.5 per 1000 for collective United States Indian groups, to 50.9% for Pima Indians in the southwest United States [24].

The American Diabetes Association recommends that children ≥85th percentile for BMI, who have any two additional risk factors (ethnic minority, positive family history, signs of insulin resistance [AN, hypertension, polycystic ovary syndrome]) be tested for glucose tolerance [30]. Recognition of T2DM is difficult in young people, and it may remain undiagnosed for a period of time. It may manifest finally as ketoacidosis, and thereby be mistaken as type 1 diabetes mellitus [30]. The pancreas in a child or adolescent may be able to produce high amounts of insulin for prolonged periods, so symptoms of overt diabetes are not present, even in the presence of gross hyperinsulinemia and IGT. In one study, 25% of obese children had IGT as measured on a 2-hour oral glucose tolerance test [31].

Etiology

What causes the cascade of events that leads to T2DM in youth? Just as there are many contributors to a cascading waterfall that gathers momentum as it travels, there are many factors that affect rates of childhood obesity, metabolic syndrome, and T2DM.

The first major factor is genetics. The increased incidence of the conditions in youth of color was identified first in the Pima Indians of the southwest. High rates of morbid obesity and diabetes were noted in this group, and a longitudinal study was begun in the 1980s. Research has focused on this group as well as other ethnic and racial groups with high rates of diabetes. It is probable that fast progression from IGT to frank diabetes is related to genetic profile. Feedback loops, enzyme systems, and membrane receptor sites are examples of factors that may be influenced genetically [22]. Genetics can play a role in an increased propensity for obesity and by progression into metabolic syndrome and diabetes once obesity is present.

The second factor of importance is dietary intake. The United States diet tends to be high in saturated and total fat and low in fiber, fresh fruits and vegetables, and dairy products. Fast food consumption and portion sizes have increased steadily, leading to caloric intake in excess of metabolic need for many in the population. Youth are particularly fond of fast foods and sugared beverages, they commonly have busy schedules that prevent families from eating at home together, and they may have access to high-density, low-nutrient foods at school and elsewhere. Although most families have an overabundance of foods, about 16.5% of families with children experience food insecurity, or a limited or uncertain access to foods at all times [7,32]. Families with food insecurity often rely on less expensive and more easily accessible high caloric-density foods. Obesity and T2DM are much more common in families with low income, which disproportionately burdens lower socioeconomic groups with these and related health problems [7].

A third factor of importance is physical activity. Youth are increasingly inactive, using screen activities for an average of 5.5 hours daily. Even the youngest children are affected; children under 6 years of age spend, on average, about 2 hours daily on screen activities, and 26% of those under 2 years of age have television sets in their bedrooms [33]. These are alarming trends, because children having more than 2 hours of screen activities daily are 73% more likely to be at risk for T2DM [34]. Inactive pursuits do not require high-caloric energy, which leads to an imbalance in intake and demand for calories. Additionally, sedentary pursuits, such as television viewing, often are accompanied by ingestion of high-calorie "junk" foods. Many of the sedentary behaviors of youth, such as television viewing and computer use, also subject them to the effects of the media, which tends heavily toward advertisements of less healthy foods. Youth spend much of their time in schools, but even this setting has decreased the physical activity levels that were common in the past. Only 25% of youth attend physical education classes daily [35]. Most school sports teams from middle school age onward require tryouts and elimination of all but a small group of students with greater ability to meet the team needs. Other children have no opportunity for sports unless the family has the time and financial resources to join private sports clubs or youth activities.

Although clearly related to a low level of physical activity, environmental design has been implicated in contributing to physical inactivity generally and to promoting other unhealthy behaviors. Many youth live in locations with unsafe or unavailable play areas. Often, sidewalks and playgrounds are not present in neighborhoods, and busy families cannot get their children to safe areas for activities on a daily basis. Walking and bicycling to activities has become virtually unknown, for convenience and safety reasons. Usually, children are transported to school by automobile or bus, and are driven to afternoon activities or return home. Most families live in urban or suburban settings and daily physical activity is limited. Community design also has facilitated signage and ready access to fast food restaurants and drive-up eateries.

One additional factor in the development of insulin resistance is pertinent to a discussion regarding youth. Recent links have been investigated between low birth weight and adult disease, such as cardiovascular disease and T2DM. Preterm and low birth weight infants have disorders in glucose control, exhibiting hypo- and hyperglycemia in the newborn period. Undernutrition in fetal life and early infancy predispose individuals to faulty cell development, "thrifty" metabolism to use all available nutrients, and enhanced stress response. All of these factors may influence development in ways that favor the development of insulin resistance, obesity, and other health consequences [36,37].

Management of obesity, metabolic syndrome, and type 2 diabetes mellitus and the nursing role

Obesity and its related problems have been identified as rampant for youth; therefore, research has begun to focus on interventions to stem and reverse the epidemic. To date, efforts have been largely unsuccessful but some hopeful trends have been identified. Experts now believe that multifaceted strategies are needed for effective outcomes [7]. To staunch a cascading waterfall, a variety of approaches can be used. A dam can be placed near the top, a series of culverts can be placed to redirect any water that escapes, diversion of contributing streams can be used, and a plan for diversion of rainwater can be devised. Likewise, strategies to deal with the epidemic of youth obesity and related outcomes should apply numerous approaches simultaneously. Nurses are key health care professionals in identifying and applying these various strategies. Individual children are targeted, especially when they exhibit some risk factors. Groups of children are the focus of population-based approaches in school systems and communities. Families are targeted so that all family members can learn about and set goals related to improved health. Schools are key components in intervention for children because so much of the day is spent in that setting. Communities bear a responsibility for providing a setting where children can be safe and healthy.

Prevention and early identification

The first major approach involves prevention and early identification of the problem. This strategy can be implemented in all settings where children are seen. For example, the adolescent who is hospitalized for an orthopedic surgery, the child seen in a clinic for asthma, or the school child who visits the school nurse office with a health problem all may be overweight and have related health problems. Astute observations and use of succinct history forms can provide valuable data to identify obesity.

A family and demographic history provide data about risk. Family history of diabetes, overweight, hypertension, and cardiovascular problems should be taken. Between 45% and 80% of youth who have T2DM have at least one parent who has diabetes, and 74% to 100% have a first- or second-degree relative who has diabetes [30]. Being part of an ethnic or racial group with a high incidence of obesity and T2DM is informative. Native Americans, Alaska Natives, Hispanics, African Americans, and Asian/Pacific Islanders are at increased risk. If ethnic group is accompanied by family history and other risks, such as obesity, referral or further testing may be warranted.

Another key component of early identification is body measurement. Height, weight, and calculation of BMI and BMI percentile should be done on individual children in all health care settings [38]. A Web-based course to teach BMI calculation and percentile analysis is available through the Centers for Disease Control and Prevention [39]; BMI percentile charts also are available through this Web site. Further assessment of body measurement, such as waist circumference or skinfold evaluation, may be appropriate in certain settings to provide additional data about individual children. For example, in an adolescent who is muscular, the BMI percentile may be deceivingly high, and additional studies may help to identify the youth who has high muscle mass but normal fat mass. In addition to individual measurements, nurses can be active in population-based programs, such as school screenings, to be sure that measurements are obtained accurately, BMI is calculated, and follow-up for abnormalities occurs. Several states, such as New York, Illinois, and Arkansas, have implemented screenings of large cadres of school children, and have used the epidemiologic data to inform the nutrition and activity programs of their schools and communities.

Nurses are instrumental in these efforts and can lead the programs, as well as serve on committees to plan for school nutrition and activity programs.

BP is an additional critical body measurement of importance as a marker of metabolic syndrome. Although child and adolescent BP is measured often in clinical settings, usually it is not placed on charts to determine its percentile. Nurses should obtain and use the BP percentile charts from the National Heart, Lung, and Blood Institute [40] that display the 90th and 95th percentiles for systolic and diastolic BP for children of given age, gender, and height percentile groups [38,41]. Elevated BP always should be referred for treatment and follow-up, and the intervention should involve weight control if this also is identified as an abnormality.

The neck and other skinfolds should be observed for AN, particularly in children who are obese and have other risk factors. AN is ranked from 0 to 4 for severity in neck and axilla neck texture, and for presence or absence on knuckles, elbows, and knees [42]. In some cases, the child will have a fasting blood draw for lipids, glucose, and insulin. These values always should be considered in the early identification of metabolic problems. Elevated triglycerides (≥ 150 mg/dL for children), low HDL-C (< 40 mg/dL for children), and elevated glucose (≥ 100 mg/dL for children) are indicative of metabolic syndrome. Additionally, a lipid profile provides total cholesterol (170–200 mg/dL is borderline for children and > 200 mg/dL is high) and low-density lipoprotein cholesterol (≥ 110 mg/dL is borderline for children and > 130 mg/dL is high) [43]. Serum glucose and glucose tolerance tests are needed when children and adolescents demonstrate risks for, or symptoms of, T2DM. A casual plasma glucose of at least 200 mg/dL, a fasting plasma glucose of at least 126 mg/dL, or a 2-hour postglucose tolerance test with plasma glucose of at least 200 mg/dL is indicative of diabetes [44].

Physical activity and sedentary behaviors are associated closely with obesity and its related disorders, so all children in settings that focus on health promotion should be evaluated for physical activity levels. Several easy tools are available, such as the Leisure Time Exercise Questionnaire and the Previous Day Physical Activity Recall [45,46]. Any child who gets no strenuous activity, engages in screen activities for more 2 hours daily, or does not get at least 60 minutes of physical activity at least 5 days/week should be considered at high risk.

Lastly, the nurse must be astute in identifying youth who have T2DM, realizing that some children present with classic signs of type 1 (polyuria, polydipsia, polyphagia with fatigue and weight loss), whereas others have no overt symptoms, but manifest with associated signs (eg, obesity, hypertension, polycystic ovarian disease, menstrual irregularities) [47].

Intervention

A variety of interventions to decrease obesity and its related health problems is being tested among youth. School programs, community interventions, and individual programs for families are examples of approaches [7]. Lifestyle intervention programs with youth and their families is one approach that shows promise for stemming the cascade of health problems [48]. Intervention for control of obesity and its related disorders of metabolic syndrome and T2DM should be aimed at populations at risk, as well as tailored to individual children and families with existing health issues.

Multiple sources of information about nutrition needs of youth should be offered to families. Nurses in all settings can be involved in individualized teaching, providing brochures and posters, and recommending useful Web sites. Ideas about healthy and easy-to-prepare snacks and meals are needed. Foods to avoid or limit and substitutions should be provided. Ethnic and cultural intake should be investigated and these foods built into the food plan or nutritious alternatives provided when fat intake is high. For example, many Hispanics have high intake of cheese in native foods, but usually are willing to use low-fat cheeses when this alternative is discussed. Because families with food insecurity and low financial resources are at greater risk for obesity, ask if the family has days of the month when there is not enough food available for members of the family. Provide lists of healthy foods and snacks, food banks, summer food programs, and other resources to all families in need, or those who may know of other families who would benefit from this information.

Nurses are active in assisting school districts to improve nutrition content of school meals and to limit or eliminate vending options and sugared beverages in schools. Such population-based approaches are showing promise and need to be continued and enhanced with carefully designed research to demonstrate effectiveness. Recommending substitutes for sugared beverages that are viewed positively by youth can assist schools in continuing to sell beverages, and, thereby, enjoy the financial benefits of such sales.

Weight management is needed for children who are already above the 85th percentile for BMI. If no other risk factors are identified, maintenance of present weight while the child grows in height is recommended. The goal is achieved through nutrition and activity alterations, with regular follow-up to monitor progress. For the child from 2 to 7 years of age who is above the 95th percentile for BMI and has associated complications, weight loss may be needed, but should be no greater than 1 pound/month. For obese children older than 7 years of age, and especially those with a BMI greater than 35 kg/m^2, dietary intervention is needed often to ensure weight loss. The desired goal is a BMI less than the 85th percentile [2]. The diet recommended for children should focus on lowering total fat to 30% or less of caloric intake and saturated fat to 10% or less of caloric intake, because insulin resistance is correlated positively with dietary fat intake [49]. Fresh fruits and vegetables are emphasized to increase dietary fiber, provide antioxidants, and maintain a more uniform plasma glucose level.

Children who are diagnosed with T2DM need careful management by an endocrine specialist. Treatment may need to include medications, at least initially, to provide for glycemic control. Insulin is required for treatment of ketoacidosis and sometimes for obtaining initial control of serum glucose [50]. Metformin is approved for use in children by the Food and Drug Administration; other antidiabetic drugs are not approved for these age groups, but a few (eg, second-generation sulfonylureas [glipizide, plyburide, glimepiride], meglitinides [mitiglinide, repaglinide, nateglinide], α-glucosidase inhibitors [acarbose and miglitol], and thiazolidinediones [tosiglitazone and pioglitazone]) have been used clinically [44].

Physical activity intervention should involve all children and their families in multiple settings. Exercise increases glycogenesis and glucose uptake by the liver, glucose uptake and mitochondrial enzyme activity, and fatty acid oxidation in skeletal muscle, and, thereby, decreases visceral adiposity [49]. Screen activities should be discouraged for children younger than 2 years of age, limited to no more than 2 hours daily for children older than 2 years, and children should never have television, computers, and other screen access in their bedrooms [51]. Nurses ask about access to sports in school, neighborhood, and the community, and provide resources as needed. Families should be encouraged to find activities that they can do together, as well as ways to foster individual physical activity interests. Suggestions for ways to increase activity on a regular basis, such as taking stairs, parking far from the supermarket door, and walking to friends' houses when it is safe to do so, are useful for families. Nurses also play a key role in population-based approaches to physical activity by working within schools as they establish physical activity plans, by helping teachers to integrate physical activity into classrooms, and by assisting with after-school activity programs. Students should have at least 30 minutes of moderate to vigorous activity daily at school, intramural and club sports should be available to all, and schools should work to promote programs for walking and bicycling to school [7].

Evaluation

Programs must be evaluated for efficacy. Concrete measurement of desired outcomes, such as BMI percentile, BP, serum lipid profile, serum glucose or insulin, self-concept and depression scores, physical activity parameters, school programs, and community characteristics, are examples of outcomes for individuals that can and should be tested. In addition, population-based evaluations are needed. These may reflect the incidence of children in a particular clinical setting, school, or community who exceed the 85th percentile for BMI or the 90th percentile for BP. Dietary evaluation of school meals and environment assessments provide further evaluative data for communities.

Summary

Countries in North America and throughout the world have become the home for a cascading waterfall of events, leading from childhood obesity to multiple health problems. The flow can be interrupted by lifestyle modifications and weight control in childhood [52–54]. Health care professionals must perform thorough assessments of children in a variety of settings, identify individuals and populations at risk, apply preventive strategies, and implement multifaceted interventions for obese youth with related health problems.

References

[1] American Academy of Pediatrics. Prevention of pediatric overweight and obesity. Pediatrics 2003;112:424–30.
[2] Centers for Disease Control and Prevention. Overweight children and adolescents: Recommendations to screen assess and manage. Available at: http://www.cdc.gov/nccdphp/dnpa/growthcharts/training/modules/module3/text/intro.htm. Accessed on June 23, 2006.
[3] National Center for Health Statistics. QuickStats: prevalence of overweight among children and teenagers, by age group and selected period – United States, 1963–2002. Morb Mortal Wkly Rep 2005;54:203.
[4] Centers for Disease Control and Prevention. Obesity is still a major problem. Available at: http://www.cdc.gov/nchs/pressroom/06facts/obesity03_04.htm. Accessed June 22, 2006.
[5] Anderson PM, Butcher KF. Childhood obesity: trends and potential causes. Future of Children 2006;16(1):19–45.
[6] Mason J, Meleedy-Rey P, Chrisoffel KK, et al. Prevalence of overweight and risk of overweight among 3- to 5-year-old Chicago children, 2002–2003. J Sch Health 2006;76(3):104–10.
[7] Institute of Medicine. Preventing childhood obesity. Washington, DC: National Academies Press; 2005.
[8] Reaven GM. Banting Lecture 1988: role of insulin resistance in human disease. Diabetes 1988;37:1595–607.
[9] Zimmet P, Magliano D, Matsuzawa Y, et al. The metabolic syndrome: a global public health problem and a new definition. J Atherscler Throm 2005;12:295–300.
[10] Bindler RM, Massey L, Shultz JA, et al. Metabolic syndrome in a multiethnic sample of school children: Implications for the pediatric nurse. J Pediatr Nurs, in press.
[11] Golley RK, Magarey AM, Steinveck KS, et al. Comparison of metabolic syndrome prevalence using six different definitions in overweight pre-pubertal children enrolled in a weight management study. Int J Obes 2006;30:853–60.
[12] Duncan GE, Li SJ, Zhou XH. Prevalence and trends of a metabolic syndrome phenotype among US adolescents, 1999–2000. Diabetes Care 2004;27:2438–43.
[13] Cook S, Weitzman M, Auinger P, et al. Prevalence of a metabolic syndrome phenotype in adolescents. Arch Pediatr Adolsec Med 2003;157:821–7.
[14] Invitti C, Maffeis C, Gilardini L, et al. Metabolic syndrome in obese Caucasian children: prevalence using WHO-derived criteria and association with nontraditional cardiovascular risk factors. Int J Obes 2006;30:627–33.
[15] Shils ME, Shike M, Ross AC, et al. Modern nutrition in health and disease. 10th ed. Philadelphia: Lippincott Williams & Wilkins; 2005.
[16] Scott LK. Insulin resistance syndrome in children. Pediatr Nurs 2006;32(2):119–25.
[17] Weiss R, Dzuira J, Burgert T, et al. Obesity and the metabolic syndrome in children and adolescents. N Engl J Med 2004;350(23):2362–74.

[18] Weiss R, Caprio S. Altered glucose metabolism in obese youth. Pediatric Endocr Rev 2006;3: 233–8.

[19] American Diabetes Association. Clinical practice recommendations. Diabetes Care 2005;28: S1–79.

[20] Reaven GM. The insulin resistance syndrome: definition and dietary approaches to treatment. Annu Rev Nutr 2005;25:391–406.

[21] Centers for Disease Control and Prevention. CDC statement on screening children for acanthosis nigricans in schools and communities. 2005. Available at: http://www.cdc. gov/ diabetes/news/docs/an.htm. Accessed June 22, 2006.

[22] Gunger N, Hannon T, Libman I, et al. Type 2 diabetes mellitus in youth: the complete picture to date. Pediatr Clin North Am 2005;52(6):1579–609.

[23] Narayan KM, Boyle JP, Thompson TJ, et al. Lifetime risk for diabetes mellitus in the United States. JAMA 2003;290:1884–90.

[24] Fagot-Capagna A, Pettitt DJ, Eneelgau MM, et al. Type 2 diabetes among North American children and adolescents: an epidemiological review and a public health perspective. J Pediatr 2000;136:664–72.

[25] Goran MI, Ball GD, Cruz ML. Obesity and risk of type 2 diabetes and cardiovascular disease in children and adolescents. J Clin Endocrinol Metab 2003;88(4):1417–27.

[26] Davis J, Busch J, Hammat A, et al. The relationship between ethnicity and obesity in Asian and Pacific Islander populations. A literature review. Ethn Dis 2004;14(1):111–8.

[27] Fagot-Campagna A, Saadine JB, Flegal KM, et al. Diabetes, impaired fasting glucose, and elevated HbA1c in US adolescents: The Third National Health and Nutrition Examination Survey. Diabetes Care 2001;24(5):834–7.

[28] Centers for Disease Control and Prevention. Diabetes projects. 2005. Available at: http:// www.cdc.gov/diabetes/projects.cda2.htm. Accessed June 23, 2006.

[29] Centers for Disease Control and Prevention. Fact sheet: trends in diabetes prevalence among American Indian and Alaska Native children, adolescents, and young adults – 1990–1998. Available at: http://www.cdc.gov/factsheets. June 23, 2006.

[30] American Diabetes Association. Type 2 diabetes in children and adolescents. Pediatrics 2000;105(3):671–80.

[31] Sinha R, Fisch G, Teague B. Prevalence of impaired glucose tolerance among children and adolescents with marked obesity. N Engl J Med 2002;346(11):802–10.

[32] Nord M, Andrews M, Carolson S. Household food security in the United States, 2002. Alexandria (VA): USDA Economic Research Service. Food Assistance and Nutrition Research Report 35; 2003.

[33] Rideout VJ, Vandewater EA, Wartella EA. Zero to six: electronic media in the lives of infants, toddlers and preschoolers. Menlo Park (CA): Kaiser Family Foundation; 2003.

[34] Urrutia-Rojas X, Menchaca J. Prevalence of risk for type 2 diabetes in school children. J Sch Health 2006;76(5):189–94.

[35] United States Department of Health and Human Services. Physical activity and health: a report of surgeon general executive. 1999. Available at: http://www.cdc.gov/ncckphp/sgr/pdf/ execsumm.pdf. Accessed June 1, 2006.

[36] Barker DJP. The developmental origins of insulin resistance. Horm Res 2005;65(Suppl 3): 2–7.

[37] Mericq V. Prematurity and insulin sensitivity. Horm Res 2006;65(Suppl 3):131–6.

[38] Bindler RM, Bruya MA. Evidence for identifying children at risk for overweight, cardiovascular disease, and type 2 diabetes in primary care. J Pediatr Health Care 2006; 20(2):82–7.

[39] Centers for Disease Control and Prevention. Available at: http://www.cdc.gov.nccdphp/ dnpa/growthcharts/guide.htm. Accessed on December 1, 2006.

[40] National Heart, Lung, and Blood Institute. Available at: www.nhlbi.nih.gov/health/prof/ heart/hbp/hbp_ped.pdf. Accessed on December 1, 2006.

[41] National High Blood Pressure Education Program Working Group on High Blood Pressure in Children and Adolescents. The fourth report on the diagnosis, evaluation and treatment of high blood pressure in children and adolescents. Pediatrics 2004;114:555–76.

[42] Burke JP, Hale DE, Hazuda HP, et al. A quantitative scale of acanthosis nigricans. Diabetes Care 1999;22:1655–9.

[43] Kavey RE, Daniels SR, Lauer RM, et al. American Heart Association guidelines for primary prevention of atherosclerotic cardiovascular disease beginning in childhood. Circulation 2003;107:1562–6.

[44] Copeland KC, Chalmers LJ, Brown JD. Type 2 diabetes in children: oxymoron or medical metamorphosis? Ped Annals 2005;34(9):686–97.

[45] Sallis JF, Buono MJ, Roby JJ, et al. Seven-day recall and other physical activity self-reports in children and adolescents. Med Sci Sports Exerc 1993;25:99–108.

[46] Weston AT, Petosa R, Pate RR. Validation of an instrument for measurement of physical activity in youth. Med Sci Sports Exerc 1997;29:139–43.

[47] McKnight-Menci H, Sababu S, Kelly SD. The care of children and adolescents with type 2 diabetes. J Pediatr Nurs 2005;20:96–106.

[48] Monzavi R, Dreimane D, Geffner ME, et al. Improvement in risk factors for metabolic syndrome and insulin resistance in overweight youth who are treated with lifestyle intervention. Pediatrics 2006;117:1111–8.

[49] Artz E, Freemark M. The pathogenesis of insulin resistance in children: metabolic complications and the roles of diet, exercise and pharmacotherapy in the prevention of type 2 diabetes. Pediatr Endocrin Rev 2004;1:296–309.

[50] Berry D, Urban A, Grey M. Management of type 2 diabetes in youth (Part 2). J Pediatr Health Care 2006;20:88–97.

[51] American Academy of Pediatrics, Committee on Public Education. Children, adolescents, and television. Pediatrics 2001;107:423–6.

[52] Berry D, Urban A, Grey M. Understanding the development and prevention of type 2 diabetes in youth (Part 1). J Pediatr Health Care 2006;20:3–10.

[53] Steinberger J, Daniels SR. Obesity, insulin resistance, diabetes, and cardiovascular risk in children. Circulation 2003;107:1448–53.

[54] Sturm R. Childhood obesity – what we can learn from existing data on societal trends. Part 1. Preventing chronic disease. Available at: http://www.cdc.gov/pcd/issues/2005/jan/04_0038.htm. Accessed on June 23, 2006.

ELSEVIER
SAUNDERS

NURSING
CLINICS
OF NORTH AMERICA

Nurs Clin N Am 42 (2007) 43–57

Diabetes Update: Injectable Therapies for Type 2 Diabetes: Practical Applications for Older Adults With Pancreatic Failure

Ginger Raterink, DNSc, ANP-C

*University of Colorado Health Sciences Center, School of Nursing, Campus Box C288-19,
4200 East 9th Avenue, Denver, CO 80262, USA*

Diabetes mellitus is a recognized epidemic in the United States. The prevalence exceeds 20 million people, with most of those having the type 2 form. Complications involve micro- and macrocirculation, with cardiovascular disease representing the leading cause of death. In addition to overt diabetes, an alarming number of people have been diagnosed with metabolic syndrome within the last few years. More than 24% of the United States population has been diagnosed with this syndrome.

As the population gets older, the natural aging process results in gradual pancreatic failure that creates challenges to the management of older adults who have type 2 diabetes. Many of this population, who experience failure of the pancreas, no longer respond to current oral regimens. Injectable therapies, particularly insulins, become necessary management tools to maintain glycemic control and to reduce the complications that are associated with micro- and macrovascular disease. This article presents a brief overview of the normal and pathophysiologic mechanisms. Introduction to management options, particularly using injectable therapies, is discussed based on the pathophysiology; it is followed by guidelines for conversion to, and management of, therapies using injectable medications.

Glucose metabolism: normal and altered physiology

Normal physiology of glucose metabolism begins with insulin, which is produced by the beta cell of the pancreas. Because the pancreas is an

---

E-mail address: ginger.raterink@uchsc.edu

0029-6465/07/$ - see front matter © 2007 Elsevier Inc. All rights reserved.
doi:10.1016/j.cnur.2006.11.003

endocrine gland that produces hormones and an exocrine gland that produces digestive enzymes, it is responsible for much of the metabolism of glucose that occurs in the body. The pancreas is the site of the islet cells of Langerhans. These cells secrete glucagon (alpha cells) and insulin (beta cells). The islets also contain delta cells that secrete somastatin, which is involved in carbohydrate, protein, and fat metabolism, probably through regulation of the α and beta cells [1].

Insulin is synthesized from proinsulin, which is composed of A peptide and B peptide connected by C peptide. Insulin is derived from the A and B peptides, which release the C peptide as the newly formed insulin hormone is released into circulation. Insulin secretion is stimulated by changes in blood glucose, amino acid and free fatty acid levels, and gastrointestinal hormones indirectly and directly through parasympathetic stimulation of the beta cells. The major function of insulin is the facilitation of glucose uptake into all cells of the body, but specifically the liver, muscle, and adipose tissue [1].

Glucagon, the other major pancreatic hormone, works antagonistically with insulin functioning to stimulate endogenous glucose formation when exogenous glucose levels decrease. Glucagon is formed by the α cells in the pancreas, as well as cells along the gastrointestinal lining. Sympathetic stimulation and circulating amino acids increase the amount of glucagon secretion, which, in turn, stimulates the liver and muscle to produce glucose [1].

Type 2 diabetes results when there are inadequate quantities of insulin in the circulation to facilitate cellular glucose transport. The consequence is an elevated level of serum glucose or hyperglycemia. The effects of elevated glucose initially involve stimulation of the pancreas to secrete more insulin. Over time, the pancreas is not able to accommodate this increased need, and glucotoxicity ensues. Patients only experience symptoms when the level of circulating glucose continues to increase and interferes with normal organ function. At this point, patients feel the increased hunger from a relative intracellular hypoglycemia that signals the brain to encourage increased glucose intake. Because of the increased amount of large glucose molecules in the blood, osmotic diuresis occurs, which causes a relative decrease in circulatory volume and an increase in urine output. Indirectly, the decreased volume signals the brain to retain water, and, in turn, stimulates the thirst mechanism [2].

The problem of insufficient insulin secretion is only part of the picture. A second mechanism for hyperglycemia was recognized recently as contributing to poor glucose to cell transport. This mechanism involves a process of resistance between circulating insulin and glucose [2]. The exact mechanism for this resistance is unclear; however, recent studies have suggested a role of adipose tissue in this process. What is known is that adipose tissue is an endocrine gland that is responsible for several hormones that control hunger, satiety, and metabolism. When the adipose tissue enlarges, its normal function is interrupted, which results in decreased levels of hormones. One hormone in particular that seems to play a role is adiponectin. In the body, adiponectin facilitates increased fat oxidation, improves insulin action in the liver and skeletal muscle, and demonstrates antiatherogenic characteristics. When adiponectin levels are decreased because of fat cell dysfunction, the liver generates glucose at accelerated levels and skeletal muscle uses glucose less well; these lead to overproduction of glucose and an imbalance of, or resistance to, the insulin–glucose connection [3].

Another process that contributes to the imbalance of glucose to insulin involves the glucose-stimulated release of insulin. Normally, the beta cell responds to a rapid glucose influx by secreting a significant amount of insulin, designed to accommodate the increased serum glucose. This is called the first-phase insulin release [2]. Once the initial glucose influx is complete and a gradual decline in exogenous glucose ensues, liver and muscle respond by releasing a consistent flow of endogenous glucose. The beta cell continues to secrete insulin on a more gradual slope, increasing as more endogenous glucose is formed and presented in the circulation (second-phase insulin release). This two-phase process represents the normal physiologic response of insulin to serum glucose elevations. In the diabetic patient, release of insulin in response to glucose stimulation changes so that the first-phase insulin surge is blunted. In part, this change signals the relative demise of the beta cell, because it no longer provides adequate amounts of insulin during the first-phase glucose increase. There remains a gradual release (second phase), although this too can be blunted as the beta cells die and the pancreas fails to function [1].

Regardless of the mechanism, the result is too much glucose for the available circulating insulin. As the beta cell attempts to accommodate larger amounts of glucose, it reaches a point where it can no longer meet the needs. The result is a gradual progressive replacement of beta cells by amyloid. This process of programmed cellular death is known as apoptosis. As the amount of active beta cells declines, there is a continual relative hyperglycemia that ultimately overpowers the beta cell and fosters the progression of amyloid replacement and apoptosis. At this point, therapies that rely on some beta-cell function are no longer effective in managing diabetes, and replacement therapies must be considered. Studies have suggested that the process of apoptosis may be reversible if glucose levels are reduced through careful medical management using injectable insulin earlier in the management process [4]. Understanding these pathophysiologic mechanisms can guide the clinician to make management decisions that will delay these processes and provide better care for the diabetic patient. Fig. 1 summarizes these mechanisms for impaired glucose metabolism and symptomatic response.

Therapeutic options

Considering the pathophysiologic processes described above, management initially was directed toward stimulation of the pancreas to secrete

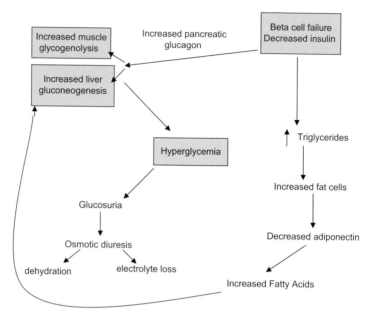

Fig. 1. Mechanisms of hyperglycemia.

more insulin. The approach was to use oral agents known as secretagogues or sulfonylureas. With further understanding of the various pathophysiologic mechanisms for glucotoxicity, oral agents directed to correct the insulin resistance and hepatic glucose overproduction have been developed. The biguanide Metformin and the thiazolidinediones work at different sites within the body to stimulate sensitivity to insulin at the cell membrane. These agents are effective in improving glucose control through a better internal use of insulin. Metformin has the added benefit of promoting weight loss and improved lipid profiles. The thiazolidinediones are the most effective insulin sensitizers in that their action improves glucose responsiveness in the skeletal muscle cells, fat, and liver. In addition, they reduce hepatic glucose production through a mechanism that—although not fully understood—seems to promote binding of the drug with receptors that are involved with glucose and lipid metabolism [5].

A final class of oral agents is the α-glucosidase inhibitors. This group of drugs acts in the gut to delay the absorption of carbohydrate. By delaying the phase 1 postprandial glucose surge, there is a reduction in the initial stimulus to the pancreas to release insulin. In so doing, the imbalance of glucose to insulin is not as severe, which allows the pancreas to maintain a level of insulin secretion that is sufficient to meet the cellular needs [6].

By the time symptoms of type 2 diabetes appear, it is estimated that only 50% of the beta cells are still functioning. The United Kingdom Prospective Diabetes Study (UKPDS) [7] demonstrated that as the disease progresses, so does the deterioration of the beta cell. This occurs despite diet, exercise, or medications. Efforts to understand this process in the body have focused on ways of measuring serum insulin levels. It is known that insulin secretion, as a measure of beta-cell function, is difficult to obtain because of the pulsatile secretory pattern. When A and B peptides combine to form insulin, they remain attached to the C peptide. Understanding this process, efforts directed toward measurement of insulin secretion indirectly through C peptide measures have been developed; however, the presence of a low C peptide level may reflect beta-cell apoptosis or may be the result of glucose toxicity. Therefore, reliance on this measure to assess beta-cell viability is inaccurate at best [7]. Treatment aimed at restoration of normal beta-cell function through exogenous insulin administration seems to be the most appropriate method of returning the normal phased physiologic response to glucose and to reduce the effects of glucose toxicity.

Use of insulin in the therapy of patients who have type 2 diabetes includes three approaches. The first is augmentation, during which insulin preparations are used to augment the actions of the oral agents. A second approach involves replacement, where exogenous insulin is used to replace the function of the beta cell early in the disease process to allow beta-cell recovery, or later when the beta cell fails. A final approach involves rescue therapy and requires the short-term use of insulin during a period of uncontrolled glucose toxicity. This method is used often during the initial treatment phase when excessive glucose has been circulating for up to several years or at times of increased system stress, such as major surgeries or infectious processes. Often, there is sufficient restoration of function to allow the patient to be returned to management by oral agents alone, once the toxic effects of excessive glucose have been reversed [7].

Several insulins are on the market, with two newer forms released recently by the US Food and Drug Administration (FDA). Ultimately, the goals of therapy are to maintain an optimal level of HbA1c as a reflection of time-sensitive glucose metabolism. Results of the UKPDS suggest that patients who have type 2 diabetes require multiple therapies to maintain life-long glycemic control [8]. Therefore, providers need to understand the oral agents and their actions, the different types of insulin, and their usage in the variety of treatment situations.

Traditional forms of insulin have been categorized based on the duration of action. Newer preparations also are evaluated by this categorization; however, there has been an additional categorization based on the physiologic effect of the insulin. Insulins that maintain a basic glucose metabolism to meet the endogenous formation are known as the basal insulins. Insulins that respond to a sudden glucose load, such as after a meal, are called bolus insulins. These larger groups are subdivided by duration of action. Understanding these categories (basal versus bolus) and the effective duration of action allows the provider to use various insulins to manage augmentation, rescue, and replacement. Table 1 summarizes the available insulins.

Table 1
Insulin preparations

Insulin	Onset	Peak action	Effective duration	Maximum duration
Bolus				
Novolog	5–10 min	1–3 h	3–5 h	4–6 h
Humalog	<15 min	0.5–1.5 h	2–4 h	4–6 h
Regular (R)	30–60 min	2–3 h	3–6 h	6–10 h
Glulisine/Levamir	5–15 min	1–2 h	3–4 h	4–6 h
Basal				
NPH	2–4 h	4–10 h	10–16 h	Up to 18 h
Detemir	2–4 h	4–10 h	10–14 h	Up to 18 h
Lente	3–4 h	4–12 h	12–18 h	Up to 20 h
Ultralente	6–10 h	8–12 h	24 h	36 h
Glargine	1 h	No peak	24 h	24 h
Combinations				
70/30 NPH to Regular	30–60 min	Varies according to type	10–16 h	Up to 18 h
70/25 NPH to Lispro	15–30 min	Varies according to type	10–16 h	Up to 18 h
70/30 NPH to Aspart	10–20 min	2–3 h	24 h	24 h

Data from Refs. [7–9].

Newer insulin preparations have been developed to improve the absorption profiles. These efforts at improving the insulins available will continue to make the use of insulin in patients who have type 2 diabetes easier and more consistent with normal physiologic glucose metabolism.

A newer, injectable agent that is not an insulin drug was approved for use in late 2005. This agent, exenatide, is directed toward the control of glucoregulatory actions. The glucoregulatory actions are stimulated naturally by hormones called incretins. When incretins are secreted, the body's response is to suppress the release of glucagon from the pancreatic α cells. The results are promotion of satiety with a resulting reduction of food intake, and slowing of the rate of gastric emptying, which reduces the intestinal absorption rates of glucose. Naturally occurring incretin hormones are peptide hormones that are secreted in the small intestine in response to food intake. They also have actions within the pancreas to increase the glucose-driven insulin secretion or phase 1 secretion from the beta cells. Exenatide mimics the actions of the incretins, and is indicated as an adjunctive therapy to improve overall glycemic control. It is used as a supplement to oral agents when they do not obtain the desired control of meal-related glucose loads. The injection is enhanced by a pen delivery system, and recommendations are that patients inject the agent before the morning and evening meal for maximum effectiveness [10].

Future management options for patients who have type 2 diabetes include other new forms of insulin that are absorbed better and more accurately mimic normal physiologic responses to serum glucose levels. In addition, new delivery methods are being evaluated to allow patients more variety in how they receive their insulin medications. Such options include continuous pump systems, inhaled insulin, and continuous glucose sensors that direct the amount of insulin delivered based on intrinsic serum glucose levels [11]. Until these newer delivery systems are available, patients who have type 2 diabetes will continue to inject their medication on a scheduled basis.

Goals of therapy

Initial management of the patient who has type 2 diabetes is based on recommendations of the American Diabetes Association [12]. In general, the goals for therapy are:

Maintenance of ideal body weight
Fasting blood glucose of 80 to 120 mg/dL
Bedtime blood glucose of 100 to 140 mg/dL
Glycosylated hemoglobin less than 7%
Management of hypertension and dyslipidemia

Options for oral or injectable agents allow the health care provider flexibility in developing a regimen that maintains optimal glycemic control, reduces the risk for micro- and macrovascular complications, and fits the patient's individual needs and lifestyle. In addition, as the pancreas progresses through the aging process, the beta cells experience programmed failure or apoptosis. When this occurs, oral agents will no longer achieve the treatment goals, and insulin preparations will be required. Introduction of insulin into the regimen can be accomplished successfully using guiding principles related to the expected outcomes. Insulin therapy should be considered for all patients who have type 2 diabetes in whom glycemic control is no longer achieved. The decisions to initiate insulin therapy are based on patients' reporting of frequent blood glucose values equal to or greater than 300 mg/dL [12]. Determinations of preparations and dosages can be individualized to the patient to achieve better blood glucose control.

Guiding principles of insulin management

Decisions to initiate insulin therapy are based on the effect desired. As patients who have type 2 diabetes age, they experience organ exhaustion. Although it was shown that such exhaustion occurs in the pancreas, it also is a part of the process in the kidneys and liver. In addition, the long-term effects of hyperglycemia, even if control is close to the therapeutic goals, interfere with normal metabolism and excretion of medications, including antidiabetic oral agents. When glycemic control is no longer satisfactory with oral agents, a decision to enhance therapy with the use of insulin often is made. Goals at this point are to minimize the early morning elevated glucose. This is accomplished best with a basal insulin injection at bedtime; when the patient arises, his/her fasting glucose is close to normal. This normal baseline glucose provides an environment in which the oral agents still can be used to effectively manage food-related fluctuations of glucose throughout the day. Dosing is based on response, as measured by the early morning fasting finger stick blood sugar (FSBS). A rule of thumb is to determine body weight in kilograms, multiple by 0.5 (0.5 units/kg), and divide by 2. Thus, if a patient weighs 70 kg, the bedtime basal insulin injection could be titrated to 18 units (eg, $70 \times 0.5/2 = 18$), depending on the following morning FSBS. Another approach, using the average of several morning FSBSs, can be used to calculate the initial bedtime insulin dose. In the same 70-kg patient, begin by dividing the average of several morning fasting blood sugars by 18 or dividing the patient's body weight in kilograms by 10. Usually, beginning with 5 to 10 units in a thin, older adult is sufficient to allow the patient to adjust slowly to the new regimen. The morning fasting FSBS should be monitored carefully to determine the response and need for additional insulin. Adding by 4 units for average fasting blood sugars of greater than 140 mg/dL or 2 units for fasting blood sugars between 120 and 140 mg/dL will allow smooth transition to goal. This goal should be a fasting morning blood sugar of 80 to 120 mg/dL. At this point, the patient often is left on an oral sulfonylurea during the day to control for daytime insulin needs. If weight gain occurs, the addition of Metformin to the daily oral sulfonylurea often reduces the insulin resistance and controls for the weight gain [12]. Throughout the day, oral agents are continued with doses adjusted according to daytime preprandial and 2-hour postprandial FSBS measurements.

Over time, progressive beta-cell failure in the older type 2 diabetic patient requires insulin replacement therapy. Using the insulin preparations from Table 1, the health care provider can develop a program of basal and bolus insulin that nearly mimics normal physiology and provides better glycemic control. Older adults often view the need for replacement insulin as failure to manage their disease process. Therefore, it is important that the decision to move to an insulin replacement program be made with the patient, and be designed to accommodate individual lifestyles. If replacement therapy is initiated at the first sign of beta-cell failure, patients will discover improved health and understand the value of the decision.

The decision to move to insulin replacement therapy requires an understanding by the provider and the patient of some important concepts concerning the insulin-dosing factors, diet, exercise, and adjustment changes for special situations (eg, sick days, travel). The health care provider will first consider adding a bedtime basal insulin dosage using NPH (intermediate-acting insulin) or glargine (basal insulin). As hyperglycemia persists, bolus insulin is added at each meal to manage the phase 1 glucose surge. FSBS measurements before lunch and dinner, at bedtime, and 2 hours following the meals determine the level of control and guide decisions concerning dosing of basal and bolus insulins. Using the information obtained from these measurements, the health care provider identifies when to switch to multiple insulin injection therapy.

Patient weight is used to determine the doses of insulin to use. Total daily doses of insulin are calculated from weight and divided between bolus and basal injections. Thinner patients have a lower total daily dosage (TDD) of insulin than do heavier patients [13]. Table 2 outlines the calculated TDD.

Once the TDD is calculated, it is divided so that 50% to 60% is administered at bedtime as the basal insulin, and the other 40% to 50% is divided between meals as the mealtime bolus insulin. In the early stages, the TDD often is reduced by 10% to 20% before dividing between the basal and bolus insulins. Especially for the older adult, this reduces any likelihood of hypoglycemia as insulin therapy is initiated.

It is at this point that two key concepts need to be understood by the provider and the patient. These two concepts involve the use of the carbohydrate/insulin ratio (C:I) and the correction factor to determine dosing of bolus insulin at mealtime, as well as guiding the decisions about basal insulin. For both concepts, it is important to measure premeal and bedtime blood glucose values to determine response to therapy, as well as consider the carbohydrate content of the foods that the patient is eating.

Goals for blood sugar measurements are determined, based on the American Diabetes Association recommendations for fasting and premeal blood sugars, at values between 80 and 120 mg/dL. At bedtime, the ideal blood sugar values are 100 to 140 mg/dL. Two-hour postprandial blood sugars should be at or below 140 mg/dL to achieve good overall glycemic control [14]. Using these values as a guide, the provider and patient can determine

Table 2
Total daily insulin dose based on weight

Weight (kg)	Units of insulin/kg	Total daily insulin dose
45	0.3–.05	14–23 units
55	0.3–.05	16–27 units
64	0.3–.05	19–32 units
73	0.5–0.7	36–51 units
84	0.5–0.7	41–57 units
91	0.7–1.0	64–91 units
100	0.7–1.0	70–100 units
109	0.7–1.0	76–109 units

Newly diagnosed or thin patients should begin with 0.1–0.3 u/kg or <20 units. Patients with insulin resistance may require up to 2.0 u/kg with insulin dosage adjusted to a target blood sugar.

Courtesy of Endocrinology, Metabolism and Diabetes Practice, University of Colorado Hospital, Denver, CO.

how much insulin is needed for each meal to cover for the carbohydrate content of the meal, as well as to correct for any excessive glucose in the blood as noted by the premeal FSBS. First, it is important to understand these concepts.

The first concept is the correction factor (CF). A premeal FSBS is used to determine the starting point for serum glucose. Most patients are instructed to consider a FSBS goal of 100 mg/dL. The patient then determines how far from goal the premeal FSBS lies to calculate the dose of bolus insulin to correct for that imbalance. For example, if the premeal blood sugar is 160 mg/dL, the patient determines that it is 60 points above the goal. A predetermined calculation tells the patient how much additional insulin to take at the meal to correct for the error. This is called the CF.

The provider determines the CF factor using a standard number value and dividing by the total daily insulin dosage. This represents an estimate of how many mg/dL one unit of insulin will be needed to reduce the total blood sugar to goal. The CF is calculated using the 1650 rule; this means that the standard number value is 1650, and that value is divided by the total daily insulin dosage. If a patient's TDD of insulin is 30 units, the CF is 55 ($1650/30 = 55$). This means that 1 unit of insulin will reduce the blood sugar by approximately 55 mg/dL—for simplicity, this number is rounded up to 60. In the example above, 160 (premeal FSBS) − 100 (goal blood sugar) = 60, the patient would add 1 unit of insulin to the mealtime dose. CF is only significant for the premeal corrections; it is not used to calculate bedtime basal insulin [15].

The other key concept regarding mealtime insulin dosing, carbohydrate/insulin ratio, results from a count of the carbohydrates contained in the meal. What C:I really tells the patient is the ratio of carbohydrates in grams to the number of units of insulin required to cover that carbohydrate load and subsequent glucose surge. If used correctly, it allows the patient to adjust the insulin dosage to fit the meal, with the result that patients experience fewer highs or lows in blood sugar and better overall glycemic control. The calculation is based on the information learned in calculating the CF. If the CF determines the effect of a unit of insulin on blood sugar and the patient eats three meals a day, the CF is multiplied by 0.33 or one third (of the total meals eaten in a day). For the example above, the CF was calculated at 55 and then rounded up to 60 ($60 \times 0.33 = 19.8$ or rounded up to 20). This is the number of carbohydrates in grams that 1 unit of insulin will cover. If the patient determines the meal to contain 40 g of carbohydrates, he/she would decide on 2 units of insulin to cover the meal [15]. If we take the above example of a premeal blood sugar of 160 mg/dL, the patient would add one additional unit and take a total of 3 units for the meal.

In summary, divide 1650 by the TDD of insulin, as calculated from Table 2 and modified as discussed, to determine the CF. Use that number to add insulin to the premeal dose to correct for any elevations in FSBG above

100. In addition, multiply the CF by 0.33 to determine the C:I for each meal. Count the carbohydrates in the meal, monitor the percentage of the meal that the patient actually consumes, and make the final calculation for the premeal insulin, which is then not injected until after the meal. Remember, in older adults with smaller appetites, the key to avoiding hypoglycemic reactions from too much insulin is to calculate the actual food consumed and not what is presented to the patient. Using these formulas and calculations will help to maintain glycemic control as the patient transitions to an insulin regimen, while preventing persistent hyperglycemia and its complications.

As is clear, these are mathematic equations and concepts that are difficult to grasp for anyone, especially for the frail older adult. Initial decisions about insulin dosages often are limited to calculations based on weight alone, until the patient is accustomed to frequent FSBS checking. Then the basal and bolus insulin doses are set at a consistent level, while the patient becomes more familiar with understanding diet, carbohydrate quantities, FSBS values, and the calculations of CF and C:I. If a patient's appetite changes, as is often the case in an older adult, the calculations may result in insulin dosages that are too high. Premeal determinations of carbohydrate content need to be adjusted for total percentage of food eaten. Therefore, in directing the older adult to use these calculations, providers can guide the patient to wait to determine the final insulin dose based on the postmeal adjustment. The best rule of thumb is to calculate the total carbohydrate content before the patient eats, and then refigure using the percentage actually consumed. The insulin injection should be given at the end of the meal rather than before the meal. This accounts for variations in consumption and continues to offer coverage for what was eaten.

Carbohydrate counting

One last concept concerns the calculation of total carbohydrates contained in a meal. Before a provider can educate the patient in the use of C:I, there should be a clear understanding of carbohydrate counting for total carbohydrate meal content determination. To recall from basic nutrition, carbohydrates are the primary glucose-producing foods in the blood. They also are called starches and sugars, and, in fact, both are considered carbohydrates. These foods break down quickly after a meal, and can be measured in the blood as glucose within a few hours after consumption. Their presence in the blood after a meal creates the stimulation for insulin secretion from the pancreas during the phase 1 insulin release. Following the meal, blood levels show a sudden increase in glucose with a subsequent increase in serum insulin. Ultimately, the two join together to enter the cell membrane and provide the nutrition needed for normal cell function.

In patients who have diabetes, the goal for good nutrition is to eat a balanced meal that contains carbohydrates, proteins, and fats. The mixture depends on the level of glycemic control, as well as the overall goals for weight control. Generally, a normal balance includes 40% to 50% carbohydrates, with 25% to 30% fats, and 20% to 25% proteins. If weight loss is a goal, the adjustment includes 45 to 60 g of carbohydrates for women and 60 to 75 g for men, which means that the proteins and fats need to be reduced accordingly [12].

What foods contain carbohydrates? Starches include breads, pastas, potatoes, peas, corn, and tortillas. Sugars include the fruits, milk, and the beloved cakes, cookies, pies, and other highly sweet foods called the concentrated sugars. On many food labels, fiber is included in the carbohydrate count. Although this is an indigestible product, it is a key to proper bowel function, and actually facilitates the elimination of carbohydrate metabolism products. Some diabetic patients even notice a reduction in blood sugar when they eat foods high in fiber [15].

The key to carbohydrate counting is to learn the portion size and average carbohydrate content in grams for each of the foods eaten. Several booklets offer information on the grams of carbohydrates in such foods as the fruits, starchy vegetables, and starches. Labels on packaged foods help to determine portion size and carbohydrate content. Practice in determining the carbohydrate content will help to make this a routine process at each meal. The goal is to determine the number of carbohydrates (remember the calculation) contained in the meal, so that insulin dosage can be adjusted to cover the meal. In the previous example, the calculation resulted in a C:I ratio of 20:1. That means for every 20 g of carbohydrates the patient eats, he/she needs 1 unit of insulin. For example, a large apple contains approximately 18 g of carbohydrates and requires 1 unit of insulin. If the patient adds a slice of bread to the meal/snack, approximately 18 to 20 g of carbohydrates is added to the meal. A second unit of insulin needs to be added to cover for the two carbohydrates. Experience with individual patients will help to determine the outcome of this calculation, and allow for minor adjustments of the insulin dosage as needed to provide adequate glycemic control [15].

Some patients experience fluctuations in their postmeal blood sugars when they eat certain fats or proteins. Normally, no additional insulin is calculated for these foods, unless it is clear that they increase blood sugar higher then expected. Experience will determine if there is a consistent pattern with certain noncarbohydrate foods that require additional insulin coverage.

The concepts just discussed are the keys to success in the management of type 2 diabetes for the patient who has pancreatic *beta*-cell dysfunction and failure. These concepts are complex for many older patients to learn and understand, and they require decision making that is confusing. Consistent education, practice, and frequent follow-up will help patients adjust to these concepts. Using these concepts to approach decisions about insulin dosage will provide the older patient who experiences pancreatic decline with

Table 3
Flow chart of daily blood glucose/insulin dosage

	Date/Time														
Blood Sugar Result															
Carbohydrate consumption															
Insulin Dose/type															

diabetes management that reduces the risks for hypoglycemia and provides consistent glycemic control. This control will improve the quality of life that these older adults can enjoy.

Keeping careful records of the patient's FSBG values, insulin doses, and average carbohydrate consumptions will provide a clear picture of the responses to management. If episodes of hypoglycemia or hyperglycemia

Table 4
Blood glucose values and insulin adjustment guideline

Blood glucose	Action
High blood glucose	
Elevated early morning fasting glucose	Check blood glucose at 2–3 AM (dawn phenomenon from Somogyi effect): Glucose > 100 mg/dL increase bedtime insulin dose Switch bedtime insulin from peaking (NPH) to peakless (basal) Glucose < 70 mg/dL decrease bedtime insulin dose
High premeal glucose	Increase C:I ratio or previous meal's fixed dose
High bedtime glucose	Increase evening meal insulin
Low blood glucose	
Low early morning fasting glucose	Decrease bedtime insulin dose
Low premeal glucose	Decrease previous meal's C:I ratio or fixed insulin dose
Low bedtime glucose	Maintain bedtime blood glucose > 100 mg/dL by: Decreasing evening mealtime insulin Adding carbohydrate snack at bedtime without bolus insulin to cover, plus bedtime insulin
Low blood glucose < 70 mg/dl at any time	Treat with 15 g dextrose Adjust glucose goal to 120–180 mg/dL If caused by insulin, adjust dose down or decrease C:I ratio

Erratic glucoses may occur because of too much insulin, decreased food intake, or gastroparesis.

Courtesy of Endocrinology, Metabolism and Diabetes Practice, University of Colorado Hospital, Denver, CO.

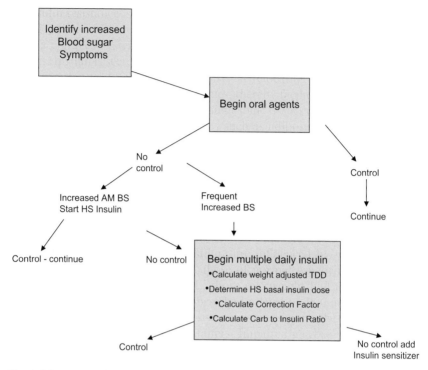

Fig. 2. Management decision points for older adults who have type 2 diabetes. BS, blood sugar; carb, carbohydrate; HS, bedtime.

occur, the provider will be able to review the records and identify possible causes for loss of control. Often, this information is best recorded on a flow chart so that results can be observed over time and patterns are identified more easily. Table 3 provides an example of a flow chart. Table 4 describes some common fluctuations in FSBS, and provides actions that can be taken to alleviate the problems. Fig. 2 depicts a summary algorithm that defines the key decision points as presented in this paper.

References

[1] McCance KL, Huether SE. Pathophysiology. The biologic basis for disease in adults and children. 5th ed. St. Louis (MO): Elsevier Mosby; 2006.
[2] Gavin JR. The pathophysiology of type 2 diabetes. Patient Care for Nurse Practitioners S 2001;4–7.
[3] Smith SR. An adipocentric view of the metabolic syndrome. Presented at the Rocky Mountain Metabolic Syndrome Symposium. Denver, CO. April 21, 2006.
[4] Kahn SE. The importance of beta-cell failure in the development and progression of type 2 diabetes. J Clin Endocrinol Metab 2001;86(9):4047–58.
[5] Porth CM. Essential of pathophysiology. Concept of altered health states. Philadelphia: Lippincott Williams & Wilkins; 2004.

[6] Blonde L. Optimizing therapy in type 2 diabetes. Patient Care for Nurse Practitioners S 2001;8–14.

[7] Mayfield JA, White RD. Insulin therapy for type 2 diabetes: rescue, augmentation, and replacement of beta-cell function. Am Fam Physician 2004;70(3):489–506.

[8] Ahmann A. A practical approach to insulin therapy in type 2 diabetes. Presented at the 2006 Rocky Mountain Metabolic Syndrome Symposium. Denver, CO. April 21, 2006.

[9] US Food and Drug Administration. FDA Consumer magazine, (January-February, 2002). Insulin preparations. Available at: www.fda.gov/fdac/features/2002/chrt_insulin.html. Accessed May 15, 2005.

[10] Barclay L. Exenatide approved for type 2 diabetes: an expert interview with John B. Buse, MD, PhD. Available at: www.medscape.com/viewarticle/504227?src=mp. Accessed May 15, 2006.

[11] Hone J. Type 2 diabetes update. Presented at the 2006 Rocky Mountain Metabolic Syndrome Symposium. Denver, CO. April 21, 2006.

[12] Mudaliar S, Edelman SV. Insulin therapy in type 2 diabetes. Endocrinol Metab Clin 2001; 30(4):1–32.

[13] McDermott MT, Dills DG. Insulin initiation and titration protocol: Endocrine, Metabolism and Diabetes Practice. Denver (CO): University of Colorado Hospital; 2002.

[14] American Diabetes Association. Diabetes Care. American Diabetes Association 1998; 21(Suppl 1):S23–31.

[15] Peralta K. Carbohydrate counting. Paper presented at the meeting on Comprehensive Diabetes Workshop. Denver, CO. July 22, 2004.

ELSEVIER
SAUNDERS

Nurs Clin N Am 42 (2007) 59–66

NURSING
CLINICS
OF NORTH AMERICA

Isolated Use of Vibration Perception Thresholds and Semmes-Weinstein Monofilament in Diagnosing Diabetic Polyneuropathy: "The North Catalonia Diabetes Study"

Jeroni Jurado, RN, DNS[a],
Juan Ybarra, MD, PhD, FACE[b],
Josep Maria Pou, MD, PhD[c],*

[a]Primary Care, Catalan Health Institute, Olot (Girona), Spain
[b]Research Institute, Hospital Sant Pau, Barcelona, Spain
[c]Department of Endocrinology, Hospital Sant Pau-Autonomous University of Barcelona,
Av. Josep Tarradellas 84-88, 2on. 1ra. 34, Barcelona 08025, Spain

Diabetic foot is a major cause of amputations in the diabetic population and its prevalence is increasing worldwide. The general consensus is that the best way to avoid this complex condition is to prevent ulcer formation [1]. Several clinical trials have demonstrated the efficacy of screening and early diagnostic strategies for diabetic polyneuropathy (DPN). Early intervention may prevent foot ulcers and amputations.

As the incidence of type 2 diabetes mellitus (T2DM) increases every year [2], it has been recommended that polyneuropathy be prevented and diagnosed at a primary care level.

Frequently, DPN diagnosis was viewed solely as a risk factor for foot ulceration, which limited the interventions to prevent possible injuries. More recently, modifiable DPN risk factors, such as metabolic control of diabetes [3], blood pressure [4], lipid profiles [5], and lifestyle [6], have been identified, and some investigations on new drugs and techniques [7,8] for its treatment

Supported by Fondo de Investigación Sanitaria (FIS), Spain. Grant number 01/0846. Spanish Network CO3/08: Instituto Carlos III.

This work was presented at the American Diabetes Association 65th Scientific Sessions. San Diego, California, June 10–14, 2005.

* Corresponding author.
E-mail address: jpou@hsp.santpau.es (J.M. Pou).

are being performed. Early detection of DPN risk would lead to a more appropriate prevention and stronger interventions on the modifiable risk factors in reversible stages of DPN.

Current evidence, however, shows that optimal screening and diagnosis methods for DPN generally are limited to cohorts in hospital centers. Simple, efficient methods are needed to perform early diagnosis of DPN and foot risk at a primary care level [9].

Several consensus reports give advice about DPN diagnosis. The San Antonio Consensus reports that at least one measurement has to be performed in five different categories [10]. Guidelines advise diagnosing DPN by the combination of different evaluations. The use of one single study has not been validated, and the predictive values are uncertain.

The authors evaluated the efficacy of the isolated use of vibration perception thresholds (VPTs) and Semmes-Weinstein monofilament (SW-MF) and compared it with a complete clinical study for DPN diagnosis.

Patients and methods

A cross-sectional prospective study of DPN diagnosis prevalence [11,12] was performed in a primary care setting in three different regions of North Catalonia (Spain), with a total population of 92,912 inhabitants. An initial random sample of 400 patients (aged 30 to 69 years) was selected, based on the reported DPN prevalence of about 30% (precision, 5%; CI, 95%) from our T2DM population from North Catalonia. Three hundred and five patients (76.75%) met the inclusion criteria (21 were lost to follow-up, 24 met exclusion criteria, 34 gave no written informed consent, 14 had other chronic illness). No difference was observed between the sample and the T2DM general population with respect to sex and age (CI: 95%).

A reference sample of 290 subjects who did not have diabetes or neuropathy was selected as a control group (CI: 95% for sex and age).

Selection criteria

Patients who had T2DM were diagnosed according to World Health Organization guidelines [13].

Exclusion criteria

Exclusion criteria included all neuropathies of other etiology, high alcohol ingestion (>60 g/d [women] and ≥ 80 g/d [men]), previous foot ulcers, and refusal to give consent.

Diabetic polyneuropathy diagnosis

Our clinical neurologic examination (reference standard) was performed based on three categories of the San Antonio Consensus for DPN diagnosis [10].

1. Neuropathic symptoms were assessed by means of modified Neuropathy Symptom Score [14].
2. Physical examination:
   Muscle strength and reflexes according to the Michigan Diabetic Neuropathy Score (MDNS) [15].
   Superficial pain sensation using sterile neurologic examination pins (Neurotips, Owen Mumford, Oxford, UK) that were applied on the dorsum of the great toe.
   Temperature perception evaluated by placing a cold tuning fork on the dorsal foot according to Young criteria [14].
3. Semiquantitative and quantitative sensory tests:
   VPTs were evaluated by two methods:
   Neurothesiometer (HORWELL Wilford Industrial). Values greater than 18 V (99th percentile in the control group) were considered to be abnormal.
   Quantitative tuning fork (Rydel-Seiffer AB-125 c64/c128) according to Liniger and colleagues [16]. Values less than 5 mgHz (5th percentile in the control group) were considered to be abnormal.
   Tactile sensitivity was measured by SW-MF 5.07/10 g (Sensifil, Novalab Ibérica). Two criteria were used, the Olmos technique [17] and MDNS [15] criteria.

VPTs (quantitative tuning fork and neurothesiometer) and SW-MF (Olmos and MDNS criteria) also were used as an isolated evaluation for DPN diagnosis. The study was performed by 12 general practitioners and 16 nurses. Clinical parameters, symptoms, and signs were evaluated by two observers. The protocol was approved by the Primary Care Ethics Board, and all participants provided written informed consent.

Data were analyzed by the SPSS Inc. 11.5 package. Qualitative variables were described as a percentage with a confidence interval. Normalization of variables was studied, and probability values were corrected without variance homogeneity. Intra- and interobserver reproducibility were evaluated. Logistic regression was performed to predict DPN presence or absence related to VPTs and SW-MF. A value of 5% ($\alpha = 0.05$) was considered to be significant.

Sensitivity and specificity for each test were analyzed by present receiver operating characteristics (ROC) curves and positive and negative likelihood ratios.

Results

DPN prevalence by our reference standard diagnosis was 23.17% (clinical neurologic evaluation). DPN prevalence by the isolated use of VPT was 14.38% and 16.34% when the evaluation was performed by neurothesiometer and quantitative tuning fork, respectively.

The prevalence by 10-g SW-MF was 9.77% with the Olmos technique and 11.40% with the MDNS technique (Table 1). DPN was significantly higher with our reference standard neurologic evaluation than with the use of isolated techniques. A high specificity (94.73% and 94.46%, respectively) and low sensitivity (43.66% and 52.11%, respectively) were observed for DPN diagnosis when neurothesiometer and quantitative tuning fork were used (Table 1).

A high specificity (95.76% and 97.88%, respectively) and low sensitivity (28.16% and 42.25%, respectively) were observed by SW-MF with the Olmos and MDNS techniques. The observed reproducibility and intra- and interassay were significant for vibration perception and MF techniques.

Quantitative tuning fork presented higher sensitivity than did neurothesiometer, and also showed more accurate positive and negative predictive values for DPN diagnosis. SW-MF evaluation of tactile sensitivity by MDNS criteria was more sensitive and showed more accurate positive and negative predictive values than did the Olmos technique.

A moderate correlation was observed between our reference standard (clinical evaluation) and quantitative tuning fork and SW-MF by MDNS; however, this correlation was significantly better for neurothesiometer than for SW-MF by the Olmos technique.

Predicted probability of DPN diagnosis was measured by the ROC curve, and it was higher with the quantitative tuning fork than with neurothesiometer and SW-MF by the Olmos and MDNS techniques (Fig. 1).

Discussion

Our clinical neurologic examination (reference standard) was established using the three categories of the San Antonio Consensus [10], and the DPN diagnosis was made after a careful evaluation of neuropathic signs and symptoms [18,19].

The results of our study showed that VPTs (performed by neurothesiometer and quantitative tuning fork) and SW-MF (by Olmos and MDNS criteria) presented high specificity and low sensitivity for DPN diagnosis in primary care settings. Nevertheless, several investigators take a single category as the "gold standard" [20,21], and they do not evaluate neuropathic symptoms.

Validity of VPTs [16,22] and SW-MF [17,23] for prediction of ulcers and amputation has been demonstrated in several studies. Despite the high specificity of these tools for ulcer risk prediction in severe DPN [24], there is no clinical evidence to support their ability to diagnose DPN when used as an isolated evaluation (without general clinical evaluation) or in the early stages of the disease [25,26].

SW-MF and VPTs are used frequently for DPN diagnosis. Their accuracy, however, has not been proven in any randomized clinical trial. These techniques show a poor correlation with the accepted traditional methods [27] and the San Antonio Consensus [10].

Table 1
Comparative studies between clinical neurologic evaluation and different techniques for diabetic polyneuropathy diagnosis in patients who have type 2 diabetes neuropathy

	CNE (Reference)	VPT-NTS	VPT-QTF	MF Olmos	MF MDNS
Prevalence	23.17%	14.38%	6.34%	9.77%	11.40%
Sensitivity	100%	43.66%	52.11%	28.16%	42.25%
Specificity	100%	94.73%	94.46%	95.76%	97.88%
Positive predictive value	100%	72.09%	74.00%	66.66%	85.71%
Negative predictive value	100%	84.37%	86.71%	81.58%	84.22%
Correct assessment	100%	82.60%	84.64%	80.13%	85.01%
Positive likelihood ratio		8.28	9.40	6.64	19.92
Negative likelihood ratio		0.59	0.50	0.75	0.59
Correlation coefficient	1	0.466	0.532	0.340	0.532
Reproducibility (CCI)					
Interobserver		0.9441 ($P < .001$)	0.8927 ($P < .001$)	Constant ($P < .001$)	0.9105 ($P < .001$)
Intraobserver		0.9747 ($P < .001$)	0.9501 ($P < .001$)	Constant ($P < .001$)	0.9720 ($P < .001$)

Abbreviations: CNE, clinical neurologic evaluation; MDNS, Michigan Diabetic Neuropathy Score; MF, monofilament; NTS, neurothesiometer; QTF, quantitative tuning fork; VPT, vibration perception threshold.

JURADO et al

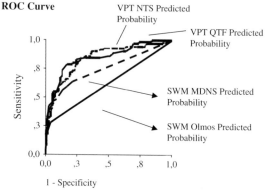

Area Under the Curve:

NTS: 0.838; QTF: 0.0847; SWM Olmos: 0.623; SWM MDNS: 0.751.

	Positive Likelihood Ratio	Negative Likelihood Ratio
VPT NTS	8.28	0.59
VPT QTF	9.40	0.50
SWM Olmos	6.64	0.75
SWM MNDS	19.92	0.59

Fig. 1. Prevalence of DPN. Sensitivity and specificity, likelihood ratio of four screening techniques. Sensitivity and specificity were plotted by ROC curve. NTS, neurothesiometer; QTF, quantitative tuning fork, SWM, SW-monofilament.

As assessments of large fiber function, the tuning fork, neurothesiometer, and MF are unable to measure small fiber dysfunction, muscle weakness, or symptoms that our gold standard assesses.

Other investigators [28–30] have found that SW-MF is a highly unreliable method for such a critical task as DPN screening. VPTs assess deep (protopathic) sensitivity, whereas DPN basically is a small fiber disease [5,31].

Although some techniques are not available at a primary care level [7,8], all diabetic patients should undergo annual screening for DPN with a complete work-up, and with the possibility to proceed with interventions for modifiable risk factors and to adapt therapy [3–6]. Prevention measures, such as intensive foot care education and diabetic treatment, should be implemented in patients who have DPN and are at risk for foot ulceration [32]. DPN screening for early detection is critical; a high sensitivity, rather than a high specificity, should be the objective.

Summary

Despite the high specificity of VPTs and SW-MF, a considerable number of patients who had DPN were not diagnosed with the isolated use of these techniques.

Acknowledgments

The authors thank Raquel Vila and Carmina Jurado, Department of Endocrinology and Nutrition, Hospital de Sant Pau, Barcelona, Spain.

References

[1] Reiber GE, Vileikyte L, Boyko EJ, et al. Causal pathways for incident lower-extremity ulcers in patients with diabetes from two settings. Diabetes Care 1999;22:157–62.

[2] Wild S, Roglic G, Green A, et al. Global prevalence of diabetes: estimates for the year 2000 and projections for 2030. Diabetes Care 2004;27:1047–53.

[3] UK Prospective Diabetes Study Group. Intensive blood-glucose control with sulphonylur-eas or insulin compared with conventional treatment and risk of complications in patients with type 2 diabetes (UKPDS 33). Lancet 1998;352:837–53.

[4] Tesfaye S, Chaturvedi N, Eaton SEM, et al, for the EURODIAB Prospective Complications Study Group. Vascular risk factors and diabetic neuropathy. N Engl J Med 2005;352: 341–50.

[5] Vinik AI, Erbas T, Stansberry K, et al. Small fiber neuropathy and neurovascular distur-bances in diabetes mellitus. Exp Clin Endocrinol Diabetes 2001;109(Suppl 2):S451–73.

[6] Smith AG, Russell J, Feldman EL, et al. Lifestyle intervention for pre-diabetic neuropathy. Diabetes Care 2006;29:1294–9.

[7] Price SA, Dent C, Duran-Jimenez B, et al. Gene transfer of an engineered transcription fac-tor promoting expression of VEGF-A protects against experimental diabetic neuropathy. Diabetes 2006;55:1847–54.

[8] Vinik AI, Bril V, Litchy WJ, et al. Sural sensory action potential identifies diabetic peripheral neuropathy responders to therapy. Muscle Nerve 2005;32(5):619–25.

[9] Boulton AJ, Vileikyte L. The diabetic foot: the scope of the problem. J Fam Pract 2000; 49(Suppl 11):S3–8.

[10] American Diabetes Association. American Academy of Neurology: Report and recommen-dations of the San Antonio Conference on Diabetic Neuropathy (Consensus Statement). Diabetes Care 1988;11:592–7.

[11] Jurado J, Bataller F, Dorca A, et al. Diabetic foot risk factors in diabetic patients with and without polyneuropathy (The North Catalonia Diabetes Study). Diabetologia 2004;47: A373–4.

[12] Jurado J, Ybarra J, Pou JM. The North Catalonia Diabetes Study (NCDS): use of vibration perception thresholds and SW monofilament for diabetic polyneuropathy diagnosis in primary care. Diabetes 2005;54:A68.

[13] Alberti KG, Zimmet PZ. Definition, diagnosis and classification of diabetes mellitus and its complications. Part 1: Diagnosis and classification of diabetes mellitus provisional report of a WHO consultation. Diabet Med 1998;15:539–53.

[14] Young MJ, Boulton AJM, Macleod AK, et al. A multicenter study of the prevalence of di-abetic peripheral neuropathy in the United Kingdom hospital clinic population. Diabetolo-gia 1993;36:150–4.

[15] Feldman EL, Stevens MJ, Thomas PK, et al. A practical two-step quantitative clinical and electrophysiological assessment for the diagnosis and staging of diabetic neuropathy. Diabe-tes Care 1994;17(11):1281–9.

[16] Liniger C, Albeanu A, Bloise D, et al. The tuning fork revisited. Diabet Med 1990;7:859–64.

[17] Olmos PR, Cataland S, O'Dorisio TM, et al. The Semmes-Weinstein monofilament as a potential predictor of foot ulceration in patients with noninsulin-dependent diabetes. Am J Med Sci 1995;309:76–82.

[18] Boulton AJM, Vinik AI, Arezzo JC, et al. Diabetic neuropathies. A statement by the Amer-ican Diabetes Association. Diabetes Care 2005;28:956–62.

[19] Boulton AJM, Gries FA, Jervell JA. Guidelines for the diagnosis and outpatient manage-
     ment of diabetic peripheral neuropathy. Diabet Med 1998;15:508–14.
[20] Adler AI, Boyko EJ, Ahroni JH, et al. Lower-extremity amputation in diabetes. Diabetes
     Care 1999;22(1):1029–35.
[21] Adler AI, Boyko EJ, Ahroni AH, et al. Risk factors for diabetic peripheral sensory neurop-
     athy. Diabetes Care 1997;20(1):1162–7.
[22] Young MJ, Breddy L, Veves A, et al. The prediction of diabetic neuropathic foot ulcerations
     using vibratory perception thresholds. Diabetes Care 1994;17:557–60.
[23] Kumar S, Fernando DJS, Veves A, et al. Semmes Weinstein monofilaments: a simple, effec-
     tive and inexpensive device for identifying diabetic patients at risk of foot ulceration. Diabe-
     tes Res Clin Pract 1991;13:63–8.
[24] Meijer JWG, Smit AJ, Lefrandt JD, et al. Back to basics in diagnosing diabetic polyneurop-
     athy with the tuning fork!. Diabetes Care 2005;28:2201–5.
[25] Kamei N, Yamane K, Nakanishi S, et al. Effectiveness of Semmes-Weinstein monofilament
     examination for diabetic peripheral neuropathy screening. J Diabetes Complications 2005;
     19:47–53.
[26] Kästenbauer T, Sauseng S, Barth H, et al. The value of the Rydel-Seifer tuning fork as a pre-
     dictor of diabetic polyneuropathy compared with a neurothesiometer. Diabet Med 2004;21:
     563–7.
[27] Mayfield JA, Sugarman JR, Peterson KA. The use of the Semmes-Weinstein monofilament
     and other threshold tests for preventing foot ulceration and amputation in persons with
     diabetes. J Fam Pract 2000;49:S17–29.
[28] Bell-Krotoski JA, Buford WL Jr. The force/time relationship of clinically used sensory test-
     ing instruments. J Hand Ther 1997;10:297–309.
[29] Booth J, Young MJ. Differences in the performance of commercially available 10-g mono-
     filaments. Diabetes Care 2000;23:984–8.
[30] McGill M, Molyneaux LM, Yue DK. Use of the Semmes Weinstein 5.07/10grm monofila-
     ment: the long and the short of it. Diabet Med 1998;15:615–7.
[31] Vinik AI, Holland MT, LeBeau JM, et al. Diabetic neuropathies. Diabetes Care 1992;15:
     1926–75.
[32] Edmonds ME, Van Acker K, Foster AV. Education and the diabetic foot. Diabet Med 1996;
     13(Suppl 1):S61–4.

ELSEVIER
SAUNDERS

Nurs Clin N Am 42 (2007) 67–78

NURSING
CLINICS
OF NORTH AMERICA

Diabetes and Depression: A Review of the Literature

Fredrick Astle, PhD, RNC

MedCentral College of Nursing, 335 Glessner Avenue, Mansfield, OH 44903, USA

Depression is a major health care condition that affects millions of people in the United States. Depression results in a major loss of work time, is a major source of hospital bed days, is one of the more disabling health care conditions, and is a leading reason for suicide. Drugs used to treat depression can lead to weight gain, which could predispose a person to type 2 diabetes; also, certain medications that may be used to treat depression with psychotic features can lead to metabolic syndrome and new-onset diabetes. Diabetes is another chronic health care condition that affects millions of people in the United States. Diabetes is the leading cause of nontraumatic amputations and a leading cause of blindness. Both conditions can result in a lower quality of life. Clinicians face challenges in treating either condition, but can face greater ones when the conditions occur together. Warren and colleagues [1] pointed out that mental illness may lead to nonadherence of treatment regimens and that "mental health problems may appear as comorbid conditions with diabetes mellitus or as complications of diabetes mellitus."

Stein and colleagues [2] found that patients who have chronic physical illnesses and comorbid depression had increased functional disability, more use of health care services, and more absences from work than did patients who had chronic physical illnesses without comorbid depression. This article reviews the literature concerning depression and diabetes.

In examining the literature, the Cumulative Index to Nursing and Allied Health Literature (CINAHL) and Proquest were used with the key words "depression and diabetes" and "diabetes and comorbid depression." Articles were included in this literature review if they addressed depression and diabetes as their primary study subject (Table 1). Articles/studies were excluded initially from review if they dealt with other issues, such as cardiovascular disease, erectile dysfunction, or studies of specific medications used to treat depression. One of the major methodological issues in

---

E-mail address: fastle@medcentral.edu

doi:10.1016/j.cnur.2006.11.007

Table 1
Presence of depression in diabetics

Study	Diabetics Controls	Gender	Age (y)	Race	Depression Assessment Method	Prevalence of Depression	Depression Scale Scores
Stein et al [2]	4.1% NC	49.3% M 50.7% F	12–50+	—	CIDI-SF	7.2%	—
Katon et al [20]	N = 4154	51.3% M 48.7% F	64.2 ± 12.6	Caucasian = 3294; African American = 350; Asian = 393; Other = 117.	PHQ-9	None, n = 3303; major, n = 497; minor, n = 354	—
Sacco et al [14]	n = 22[a] n = 34[b] NC	45% M 55% F	Mean = 54	Caucasian = 82%; Hispanic = 9%; African American = 7%; Asian = 2%.	PHQ-9	16%	Mean = 17.7[a] SD = 6.6[a] Mean = 13.4[b] SD = 4.7[b]
Kessing et al	358	31.9% M 68.1% F	43.3–68.8 Mean = 56.6	—	ICD-8 ICD-10	29.03%	—
Kessing et al	91,507 108,487	48.1% F 59.7% F	47.5–74 57.7–76.1		ICD-8	350 495	—
Bruce et al [19]	1273 NC	51.3% M 48.7% F	64.1 ± 11.2	Anglo-Celt = 61.1; South European = 16.2, Other European = 9.2; Asian = 4.5, 2.5%; Mixed/other = 7.2, indigenous Australians = 1.7, 1.1%.[c]	GHS-Q	31.5%	—

Study	N	Gender	Age	Ethnicity	Measure	Prevalence	Score
de Groot et al [17]	221 NC	39.7% M 60.3% F	53.9 ± 11.9	Caucasian = 52.9%; African American = 30.1%; Hispanic = 8.75%; Other = 8.2%.	CES-D	25.3%	32.8 ± 7.3
Blazer et al [9]	20.1[d]	65.0% F	>75 (38.9%)	African American = 54.3%	CES-D	9.6%	—
Sambamoorthi et al [18]	5%	30.7% M 69.3% F	18–64	Caucasian = 34.3%; African American = 42.7%; Latino = 3.4%; Other = 0.9%; Unknown = 18.7%.	ICD-9	10.1%[e] 7.3%[f]	—
Brown et al	32,257 59,420	52% M 48% F	Mean = 52 20–95[h]	—	ICD-9	2.9%[e] 2.8%[f]	—
Vileikyte et al [15]	484[g]	70% M 30% F		—	HADS	—	≥13[i]
Hood et al [25]	145	44% M 56% F	14.9 ± 2.3	—	CDI[j]	15.2%[k]	≥13
Trief et al [31]	1665	37.2% M 62.8% F	70.8 ± 6.6	Caucasian = 49.4%; African American = 14.9%; Hispanic = 35.2%; Other = 0.5%.	SHORT-CARE	31.7%[l] 27.8%[m]	5.7 ± 4.8[n]
Ludman et al [12]	4168	51.4% M 48.6% F	Mean = 63.5 SD = 13.21	Caucasian = 78.2%	PHQ	N = 487	—
Lawrence et al [35]	2672	48% M 52% F	Mean = 15.3; Range = 10–21	Caucasian = 67% ; African American = 10%; Hispanic = 14%; Other = 9%.	CES-D	n = 2067[o] n = 375[p] n = 230[q]	10.7 ± 8.6

(continued on next page)

Table 1 (continued)

Study	Diabetics Controls	Gender	Age (y)	Race	Depression Assessment Method	Prevalence of Depression	Depression Scale Scores
Pouwer et al [33]	3107[r]	48% M 52% F[v]	55–85		CES-D	16.9%[s] 7.8%[t]	u
Pouwer et al [16]	539		w	—	CES-D PAID		x
Tellez-Zenteno & Cardiel [10]	189	42% M 58% F	61.7 ± 12.5	—	BDI	39%[y]	≥14
Palinkas et al [13]	971	43% M 57% F	50–89	Caucasian = 100%	BDI		M = 5.2[z] M = 6.5[aa]
Roy & Roy [32]	581	41.3% M 58.7% F	Mean = 31.6[bb] Mean = 32.6[cc]	African American = 100%	BDI	27.4%	M = 10.7 SD = 9.5
Zhang et al [21]	714 9276				CES-D		
Levitt Katz et al [24]	237	37% M 63% F	dd	Caucasian = 13%; African American = 79%; Hispanic = 4.3%; Asian = 4.3%.	Interview	19.4%[ee]	—

Abbreviations: BDI, Beck Depression Inventory; CDI, Children's Depression Inventory; CES-D, Center for Epidemiologic Studies Depression Scale; CIDI-SF, Composite International Diagnostic Interview–Short Form; F, female; GHS-Q, General Health Status Questionnaire; HADS, Hospital Anxiety and Depression Scale; ICD-8, International Classification of Diseases, Eighth Revision; ICD-9, International Classification of Diseases, Ninth Revision; ICD-10, International Classification of Diseases, Tenth Revision; M, male; PAID, Problem Areas in Diabetes Scale; PHQ, Patient Health Questionnaire; PHQ-9, Patient Health Questionnaire-9; SD, standard deviation; Short-CARE, Short Comprehensive Assessment and Referral Evaluation Depression Scale.

a Refer to Depression Scale Scores column.
b Refer to Depression Scale Scores column.
c Data are for depressed and nondepressed groups, respectively.
d Diabetes was self-reported.
e Depression in diabetic patients.
f Depression in patients who did not have diabetes.

g The sample consisted of 316 participants from the United Kingdom and 168 participants from the United States.

h Mean age: United Kingdom, 61.5 ± 11.54; United States, 62.56 ± 9.82; total, 61.86 ± 10.98.

i United Kingdom, 5.41 ± 4.26; United States, 4.83 ± 3.65; total, 5.20 ± 4.06.

j Score ≥13.

k Prevalence of depression in total N, including male and female subjects.

l Score >7 yields highest specificity for depression.

m Percentage of respondents who had depression at baseline.

n Percentage of respondents who had depression at follow-up.

o Minimal score <16.

p Mildly depressed score 16–23.

q Moderately to severely depressed score ≥24.

r Seven percent (216 subjects) had type 2 diabetes.

s Prevalence of pervasive depression in all subjects who had type 2 diabetes.

t Prevalence of pervasive depression in subjects who had type 2 diabetes and no other chronic disease.

u Scores 6.0 ± 6.8 no chronic disease; 6.9 ± 7.7 type 2 diabetes only; 8.0 ± 7.1 type 2 diabetes with comorbidity (significant at P<.001).

v Croatian subjects (50% M and 50% F), Dutch subjects (55% M and 45% F), English subjects (47% M and 53% F).

w Croatian subjects (53 ± 11 M, 53 ± 15 F), Dutch subjects (54 ± 15 M, 54 ± 16 F), English subjects (57 ± 14 M, 55 ± 17 F).

x Croatian subjects (14.5 ± 11.4 M, 14.3 ± 10.9 F), Dutch subjects (8.1 ± 9.3 M, 9.7 ± 8.3 F), English subjects (11.5 ± 9 M, 15.2 ± 12 F).

y Of depressed patients, 32% had major depression (BDI ≥21) and 68% had minor depression.

z Mean score at visit 1.

aa Mean score at visit 2.

bb Mean age (SD, 9.1) for those with BDI >14.

cc Mean age (SD, 8.3) for those with BDI ≤14.

dd Mean age was 14.7 years (SD, 2.5) for those who had a neuropsychiatric disorder and 13.7 years (SD, 2.9) for those who did not have a neuropsychiatric disorder.

ee For any neuropsychiatric disorder.

the studies conducted is the lack of control groups and the wide variety of methods used to measure depression (many are self-reporting–type scales). This may lead to bias issues because persons who are medically ill may report more depression-like symptoms.

Anderson and colleagues [3] conducted a meta-analysis relating to the prevalence of comorbid depression in diabetic adults. The group analyzed 42 studies that used a nondiabetic comparison group; the presence of diabetes doubled the chances of having comorbid depression. Eaton [4], in a brief review of epidemiologic evidence regarding the comorbidity of depression and diabetes, found extensive evidence that diabetes and depressive disorder occur together more often than would be expected by chance association. Examining prospective, population-based studies revealed that a temporal order might be occurring from diabetes to depression or from depression to diabetes, depending to some extent on the type of diabetes (eg, for type 2 diabetes mellitus depression may be primary, whereas for type 1 diabetes mellitus it may be secondary). Musselman and colleagues [5], in a review of studies done from 1966 to 2003 that investigated pathophysiologic alterations related to glucose intolerance and diabetes in depressed patients, found that recent studies demonstrated that depression and its associated symptoms constitute a major risk factor in the development of type 2 diabetes and may accelerate the onset of diabetes complications. Some limitations of studies they reviewed included not looking at minority populations or the contribution of socioeconomic status. In a review of literature, Brown and colleagues [6] found strong evidence for an association between depression and the later development of medical illness. Evidence linking elevated or temporarily dysregulated cortisol secretion with these conditions is strong, although less compelling.

In a literature review of articles that looked at outcomes, relationships, and management of comorbid depression and diabetes from 1980 to 2002, Lustman and Clouse [7] found that depression is common in types 1 and 2 diabetes.

Knol and colleagues [8] conducted a meta-analysis of studies that looked at depression as a risk factor for the onset of type 2 diabetes. When they analyzed nine longitudinal studies, they found that adults who had a high risk for depression had a 37% increased risk for developing type 2 diabetes compared with those who were not depressed or had symptoms of mild depression.

Blazer and colleagues [9] explored the risk for comorbid depression/diabetes and depression/higher body mass index in older African American adults; they found significant comorbidity between depression and diabetes, although they did not characterize it as dramatic (twice what would be expected by chance). Tellez-Zenteno and Cardiel [10] found that poor compliance with different therapeutic regimens was associated strongly with the presence of depression and that diabetes mellitus is an important health issue in Mexico with medical, social, and economic impact. In a population-based sample, Carnethon and colleagues [11] found that men and women with less than a high school education who reported the highest number of symptoms of depression were at an increased risk for developing diabetes.

Ludman and colleagues [12] found that of diabetic patients, those who had major depression reported significantly more diabetic symptoms compared to participants who did not have major depression after adjusting for age, gender, marital status, education, racial ethnicity, medical comorbidities, duration of diabetes, and type of diabetes. Palinkas and colleagues [13] found in a prospective study that a depression score (Beck Depression Inventory (BDI)) of greater than 11 was associated with a twofold risk for developing type 2 diabetes 8 years later; this was consistent with two other published longitudinal studies. In addition, in older adults, depressive symptoms were more likely to be a risk factor for type 2 diabetes than the reverse.

In a study of diabetic patients recruited from a diabetes center waiting room and from a medical record search, Sacco and colleagues [14] found that less adherent patients were more depressed and had lower self-efficacy and higher body mass index. In addition, depression and obesity seemed to be risk factors for the development of type 2 diabetes. Vileikyte and colleagues [15] established an association between diabetic neuropathy and depressive symptoms. Pouwer and colleagues [16] related that depressive symptomatology was common in Croatian, Dutch, and English diabetic outpatients, serious diabetes-specific emotional problems were less common in English subjects compared with Croatian and Dutch patients (may be explained, in part, by selection bias), and diabetes-specific emotional problems were particularly common in diabetic patients who had a high level of depressive symptoms.

de Groot and colleagues [17] found that rates of depression in type 1 and type 2 diabetics were comparable to other studies (25% of which demonstrated high rates of depression compared with 25%–30% from other studies). Sambamoorthi and colleagues [18] evaluated the relationship between diabetes and depression care among nonelderly Medicaid beneficiaries; the presence of comorbid diabetes was associated with significantly higher rates of diagnosed depression.

In a study of patients who had type 2 diabetes and who did and did not have comorbid depression, Bruce and colleagues [19] found that depressed subjects were significantly more likely to have died of all causes as well as cardiac causes. Katon and colleagues [20] found that among patients who had type 2 diabetes, minor and major depression was associated strongly with increased mortality. The increased mortality in diabetics that is associated with depression is related to poor adherence to treatment regimens, poor adherence with disease control measures, and poor glucose regulation. Using survival analysis, Zhang and colleagues [21] analyzed longitudinal data from the National Health and Nutrition Examination Survey (NHANES) 1 Epidemiological Follow-up study; the presence of severe depression significantly elevated mortality risk among United States adults who had diabetes. Their findings confirmed that diabetics are prone to be depressed and that depressive symptoms play a more important role in mortality among people who have diabetes than among people who do not have diabetes.

A few studies looked at this issue in children and adolescents. In a review of the literature on the natural history and correlates of comorbid depression in children and adolescents, Grey and colleagues [22] found that the comorbidity of diabetes and depression in children and adolescents was a significant problem that affected up to 20% of youth who had diabetes, compared with less than 7% in youth who did not have diabetes. Diabetic children had a twofold greater prevalence of depression and diabetic adolescents had a threefold greater prevalence of depression than youth who did not have diabetes.

Dantzer and colleagues [23] conducted an analysis of recent literature on anxiety and depression in juvenile diabetics. The major conclusions of the review support the notion of a general association of psychologic disorders with juvenile diabetes. They related that although anxiety and depression play an important and complex role in determining adaptation to the disease, their relationship to metabolic control is not clear.

Levitt Katz and colleagues [24] found that 19.4% of youths who had type 2 diabetes had a neuropsychiatric disorder. Of these, a significant number was treated with psychotropic drugs that have been reported to cause weight gain in children and adults and to worsen type 2 diabetes mellitus in adults. Hood and colleagues [25] found that nearly one in seven diabetic youths met the clinical cutoff for depression, which was double the highest estimate of depression in youth in general. They related that this indicates the need to pay attention to emotional functioning of youth who have type 1 diabetes and to family functioning.

Not all studies postulated a relationship between diabetes and depression. Saydah and colleagues [26] conducted longitudinal analyses using data from the NHANES 1 Epidemiological Follow-up survey. They found no increased incidence of diabetes for those with high or moderate levels of depressive symptoms compared with those with no depressive symptoms. They related that these results do not support the etiologic relationship of depression predisposing individuals to diabetes. In studies done in Denmark, covering the period from 1977 to 1997, Kessing and colleagues [27,28] examined the prevalence of diabetes in persons who had depression and mania; persons who had osteoarthritis were used as the control group. Compared with controls, the risk for getting readmitted with diabetes was not increased for patients who had been admitted previously with depression. Getting a discharge diagnosis of depression on readmission showed that the risk for being readmitted with depression was no different for the diabetics compared with the control group.

In a review of published studies between 2000 and 2004, Barnard and colleagues [29] found insufficient evidence to conclude that depression is more prevalent in people who have type 1 diabetes compared with matched groups. Of 14 studies reviewed, only 4 studies concurrently examined prevalence in control groups, and only 3 studies used diagnostic interviews. They further pointed out that without a control group it is not possible to generalize study findings. In a retrospective study conducted in Canada, Brown and colleagues [30] found little evidence that type 2 diabetes increased the risk for depression once comorbid diseases and the burden of diabetes complications were accounted for. Trief and colleagues [31] found a significant correlation between depression and glycosylated hemoglobin value, which indicated that depression was associated with poor glycemic control at baseline; however, no evidence was found that depression predicts changes in glycemic control.

Four studies that were examined might be interpreted as having mixed results. Roy and Roy [32] found that more than 25% of the 581 insulin-requiring African Americans who had type 1 diabetes had a BDI (depression) score of greater than 14. They pointed out, however, that a high BDI score is not synonymous with having a major depressive episode and that the use of the BDI in medically ill patients may be problematic. They found that significantly more diabetics with a BDI score greater than 14 had proliferative diabetic retinopathy and significantly more were receiving payments for disability that was due to diabetes and its complications. Pouwer and colleagues [33] found that the odds for pervasive depression were particularly increased in subjects who had type 2 diabetes and other comorbid diseases but not in patients who had type 2 diabetes only. They further related that based on these findings and the results from other research groups, one can make the assumption that depression is a common, serious, and disabling complication of type 2 diabetes in men and women. In a review of studies, Evans and colleagues [34] found that although depression has been shown to be an independent risk factor for type 2 diabetes, methodological issues preclude definitive prevalence estimates; many studies used self-reported symptom scales that resulted in higher prevalences than when depression was determined by diagnostic interview. In addition, they found that few studies included African Americans, Native Americans, Latin Americans, children, and adolescents.

Lawrence and colleagues [35] found the following results: men who had type 2 diabetes had higher rates of moderately/severely depressed mood than did men who had type 1 diabetes; no association was found between duration of diabetes and level of depressed mood; 15.6% of men and 26.9% of women who had moderately/severely depressed mood reported being on psychiatric medication; the prevalence of mild or moderately/severely depressed mood among diabetic youth was similar to published estimates of depression prevalence among youth who did not have diabetes using the same screening tool; and depressed mood may be associated with poor glycemic control and more frequent emergency department visits.

The results of the studies reviewed are mixed—some show a relationship between diabetes and depression, whereas others have negative inconclusive results. From this, one cannot imply causation, saying that depression causes diabetes or that diabetes causes depression; however, several recommendations that were made in the studies reviewed bear repeating. Eaton [4] made a recommendation about epidemiologic studies when he stated, "epidemiological studies can help prioritize risk factors for disorders perhaps leading to efforts at prevention. The relative importance of risk factors can be estimated with population attributable risk, which is the amount that incidence can be lowered when a given risk factor is eliminated."

According to Carnethon and colleagues [11], the impact of depressive symptoms on diabetes, as reported in this study, suggests that practitioners may have an additional reason to institute targeted screening and treatment programs for depression in low socioeconomic status population. Evans and colleagues [34] and de Groot and colleagues [17] recommended that all medically ill patients be screened for depression; clinicians maintain a low threshold for depression treatment; barriers to care are identified; confront and reduce the stigma surrounding depression and bipolar disorder; expand the research agenda for bipolar disorder; focus on special populations (eg, minorities, children, and adolescents); establish a standardized database; conduct prospective, rigorously designed studies; include depression assessments in all future large-scale epidemiologic studies; and increase depression screening for ethnically diverse patients with types 1 or 2 diabetes. Ludman and colleagues [12] stated, "treating clinicians may be puzzled by patients with comorbid chronic medical conditions and depression who report higher levels of physical symptoms than other patients with comparable disease severity. High levels of symptoms that do not correlate with physical or laboratory assessments should prompt clinicians to assess for depression so that inappropriate testing or treatment recommendations are avoided."

Pouwer and colleagues [16] related that because diabetes-specific emotional problems seemed to be common, predominantly in depressed patients, health care providers who treat depression in diabetic patients should have a good knowledge about the management of diabetes, the short- and long-term complications, and diabetes-specific emotional problems. Lawrence and colleagues [35] related that health care providers should assess the history of depression among youth diagnosed with type 2 diabetes. Depression may have predated the diagnosis of diabetes, and depression may place them at increased risk for poor glycemic control and resultant health problems. Wexler [36], in a commentary, related that practitioners who care for diabetic patients are familiar with the problems of comorbid depression: decreased compliance with treatment, increased risk for complications and disability, and diminished health-related quality of life.

References

[1] Warren BH, Crews CK, Schulte MM. Managing patients with diabetes mellitus and mental health problems. administrative and clinical challenges. Disease Manage Health Outcomes 2001;9(3):123–30.

[2] Stein MB, Cox BJ, Afifi TO, et al. Does co-morbid depressive illness magnify the impact of chronic illness? A population-based perspective. Psychol Med 2006;36:587–96.

[3] Anderson RJ, Freeedland KE, Clouse RE, et al. The prevalence of comorbid depression in adults with diabetes: a meta-analysis. Diabetes Care 2001;24(6):1069–78.

[4] Eaton WW. Epidemiologic evidence on comorbidity of depression and diabetes. J Psychosom Res 2002;53:903–6.

[5] Musselman DL, Betan E, Larsen H, et al. Relationship of depression to diabetes types 1 and 2: epidemiology, biology, and treatment. Society of Biologic Psychiatry 2003;54:317–29.

[6] Brown ES, Varghese FP, McEwen BS. Association of depression with medical illness: does cortisol play a role? Biol Psychiatry 2004;55:1–9.

[7] Lustman PJ, Clouse RE. Depression in diabetic patients. The relationship between mood and glycemic control. J Diabetes Complications 2005;19:113–22.

[8] Knol MJ, Twisk JWR, Beekman ATF, et al. Depression as a risk factor for the onset of type 2 diabetes mellitus. A meta-analysis. Diabetologia 2006;49:837–45.

[9] Blazer DG, Moody-Ayers S, Craft-Morgan J, et al. Depression in diabetes and obesity. Racial/ethnic/gender issues in older adults. J Psychosom Res 2002;53:913–6.

[10] Tellez-Zenteno JF, Cardiel MH. Risk factors associated with depression in patients with type 2 diabetes mellitus. Arch Med Res 2002;33:53–60.

[11] Carnethon MR, Kinder LS, Fair JM, et al. Symptoms of depression as a risk factor for incident diabetes: Findings from the National Health and Nutrition Examination Epidemiologic Follow-up Study, 1971–1992. Am J Epidemiol 2003;158(5):416–23.

[12] Ludman EJ, Katon W, Russo J, et al. Depression and diabetes symptom burden. Gen Hosp Psychiatry 2004;26:430–6.

[13] Palinkas LA, Lee PP, Barrett-Connor E. A prospective study of type 2 diabetes and depressive symptoms in the elderly: The Rancho Bernardo Study. Diabet Med 2004;21:1185–91.

[14] Sacco WP, Wells KJ, Vaughan CA, et al. Depression in adults with type 2 diabetes: the role of adherence, body mass index, and self-efficacy. Health Psychol 2005;24(6):630–4.

[15] Vileikyte L, Leventhal H, Gonzalez JS, et al. Diabetic peripheral neuropathy and depressive symptoms. Diabetes Care 2005;28(10):2378–83.

[16] Pouwer F, Skinner TC, Pibernik-Okanovic M, et al. Serious diabetes-specific emotional problems and depression in a Croatian-Dutch-English Survey from the European Depression in Diabetes (EDID) Research Consortium. Diabetes Res Clin Pract 2005;70:166–73.

[17] de Groot M, Pinkerman B, Wagner J, et al. Depression treatment and satisfaction in a multicultural sample of type 1 and type 2 diabetic patients. Diabetes Care 2006;29(3):549–53.

[18] Sambamoorthi U, Olfson M, Wei W, et al. Diabetes and depression care among Medicaid beneficiaries. J Health Care Poor Underserved 2006;17:141–61.

[19] Bruce DG, Davis WA, Starkstein SE, et al. A prospective study of depression and mortality in patients with type 2 diabetes: The Fremantle Diabetes Study. Diabetologia 2005;48:2532–9.

[20] Katon WJ, Rutter C, Simon G, et al. The association of comorbid depression with mortality in patients with type 2 diabetes. Diabetes Care 2005;28(11):2668–72.

[21] Zhang X, Norris SL, Gregg EW, et al. Depressive symptoms and mortality among persons with and without diabetes. Am J Epidemiol 2005;161(7):652–60.

[22] Grey M, Whittemore R, Tamborlane W. Depression in type 1 diabetes in children: natural history and correlates. J Psychosom Res 2002;53:907–11.

[23] Dantzer C, Swendsen J, Maurice-Tison S, et al. Anxiety and depression in juvenile diabetes: a critical review. Clin Psychol Rev 2003;23:787–800.

[24] Levitt Katz LE, Swami S, Abraham M, et al. Neuropsychiatric disorders at the presentation of type 2 diabetes mellitus in children. Pediatr Diabetes 2005;6:84–9.

[25] Hood KK, Huestis S, Maher A, et al. Depressive symptoms in children and adolescents with type 1 diabetes. Diabetes Care 2006;29(6):1389–91.
[26] Saydah SH, Brancati FL, Golden SH, et al. Depressive symptoms and the risk of type 2 diabetes mellitus in a US sample. Diabetes Metab Res Rev 2002;19:202–8.
[27] Kessing LV, Nilsson FM, Siersma V, et al. No increased risk of developing depression in diabetes compared to other chronic illness. Diabetes Res Clin Pract 2003;62:113–21.
[28] Kessing LV, Nilsson FM, Siersma V, et al. Increased risk of developing diabetes in depressive and bipolar disorders? J Psychiatr Res 2004;38:395–402.
[29] Barnard KD, Skinner TC, Peveler R. The prevalence of co-morbid depression in adults with type 1 diabetes: systematic literature review. Diabet Med 2006;23:445–8.
[30] Brown LC, Majumdar SR, Newman SC, et al. Type 2 diabetes does not increase risk of depression. Can Med Assoc J 2006;175(1):42–6.
[31] Trief PM, Morin PC, Izquierdo R, et al. Depression and glycemic control in elderly ethnically diverse patients with diabetes. Diabetes Care 2006;29(4):830–5.
[32] Roy A, Roy MR. Depressive symptoms in African-American type 1 diabetics. Depress Anxiety 2001;13:28–31.
[33] Pouwer F, Beekman ATF, Nijpels G, et al. Rates and risks for comorbid depression in patients with type 2 diabetes mellitus: results from a community based study. Diabetologia 2003;46:892–8.
[34] Evans DL, Charney DS, Lewis L, et al. Mood disorders in the medically ill: scientific review and recommendations. Society of Biological Psychiatry 2005;58:175–89.
[35] Lawrence JM, Standiford DA, Loots B, et al. Prevalence and correlates of depressed mood among youth with diabetes: the SEARCH for Diabetes in Youth study. Pediatrics 2006;117(4):1348–58.
[36] Wexler DJ. Low risk of depression in diabetes? Would that it were so. Can Med Assoc J 2006;175(1):47–8.

NURSING
CLINICS
OF NORTH AMERICA

Nurs Clin N Am 42 (2007) 79–85

Primary Hyperparathyroidism, Insulin Resistance, and Cardiovascular Disease: A Review

Juan Ybarra, MD, PhD, FACE[a],*,
Teresa Doñate, MD, PhD[b],
Jeroni Jurado, RN, DNS[c],
Josep Maria Pou, MD, PhD[a]

[a]Servicio de Endocrinología y Nutrición, Hospital de Sant Pau, Mas Casanovas 90, Barcelona 08041, Spain
[b]Servicio de Nefrologia, Fundación Puigvert, Barcelona, Spain
[c]EAP ABS Olot, ICS. P. Barcelona s/n 17800 Olot, Girona, Spain

The presentation of primary hyperparathyroidism (PHPT) has changed substantially in the last decades. Before the introduction of routine calcium measurement in most automated biochemistry serum analyzers, it usually was diagnosed after renal and bony lesions already were present. Nowadays, its presentation is practically asymptomatic. Nevertheless, the cardiovascular morbidity and mortality of mild to moderate forms of PHPT reportedly are increasing. Individuals who have mild to moderate forms of PHPT have an increased risk for enduring cardiovascular disease, arterial hypertension (HTN), left ventricular hypertrophy (LVH), myocardial and valvular calcifications, altered vascular reactivity, and cardiac conduction. Finally, they also reveal alterations in carbohydrate metabolism, insulin resistance (IR), dyslipidemia, and body composition.

Some of these disturbances (eg, LVH, alterations in carbohydrate metabolism, IR) are reversible upon surgical cure of PHPT, whereas others (eg, HTN) persist.

In hyperparathyroidism, parathyroid hormone levels (iPTH) have been reported to have significant relationships with IR as well as several proinflammatory cytokines and clotting factors, especially in secondary hyperparathyroidism in hemodialyzed patients. IR is likely to

---

* Corresponding author.
E-mail address: juanybarra@hotmail.com (J. Ybarra).

0029-6465/07/$ - see front matter © 2007 Elsevier Inc. All rights reserved.
doi:10.1016/j.cnur.2006.11.010

be the most prominent and influential cardiovascular risk factor in this setting.

Insulin resistance

Concept

IR is defined as insulin's diminished capacity to exert its biologic actions on its target tissues (ie, skeletal muscle, liver, adipose tissue) [1]. Chronic or sustained IR is the common cause for many metabolic and nonmetabolic diseases, such as type 2 diabetes mellitus (T2DM), obesity, arterial HTN, dyslipidemia, cardiovascular disease, and cancer [2,3]. In some instances (eg, obesity), IR appears as an adaptive mechanism.

Insulin is the main anabolic and anticatabolic hormone in humans. Its principal metabolic effects are exerted on skeletal muscle, liver, and adipose tissue [4].

In skeletal muscle, insulin stimulates glucose uptake and directs it toward glycogen synthesis. Moreover, insulin reduces the hepatic production of glucose and increases the rate of glycogen synthesis. Adipose tissue is much more than a simple fatty acid storage organ. Its metabolic turnover is high, and it produces many proinflammatory adipocytokines, which are hormones with autocrine and paracrine actions. Additionally, it is the tissue where insulin antilipolytic activity is exerted, and, thus, the free fatty acid liberation into circulation is inhibited.

Insulin's antilipolytic effect accounts for more than 90% of insulin's global actions at its physiologic concentrations. Hence, insulin stimulates glucose uptake, lipogenesis, and the triglyceride depot at the adipocytes.

Measurement of insulin resistance

The euglycemic hyperinsulinemic clamp [5] is the gold standard procedure for measuring IR in small patient cohorts. It is a cumbersome procedure whose cost and difficulties have prompted research toward simpler and reproducible techniques [6,7]. Most epidemiologic studies use the HOMA index (Homeostasis Model Assessment) as a surrogate marker of IR [8]. Fasting plasma glucose and insulin are measured three times at 5-minute intervals. Their mean values are used in the following equation: glucose (mmol/L) × insulin (μUI/L)/22.5.

The HOMA formula provides a semiquantitative assessment of insulin sensitivity (as well as beta-cell function) based on structural mathematical modeling. Hence, a lean, healthy, young individual has an average of insulin sensitivity of 1 and a beta-cell function of around 100%. HOMA formula is applicable only to nondiabetic subjects.

There is great variability in insulin determination between different methods and laboratories. Hence, no standard insulin laboratory determinations have been implemented internationally. Moreover, fasting insulin concentrations have a 400% to 600% variability within subjects [7,9,10]. These considerations should be kept in mind when analyzing HOMA results.

Insulin resistance and cardiovascular risk

Epidemiologic data clearly identify IR as an independent cardiovascular risk factor [11]. Hyperinsulinemic individuals who display normal oral glucose tolerance tests (OGTTs) tend to accumulate more cardiovascular risk factor than do those with normal fasting insulin values [12]. Clinical studies suggest that myocardial perfusion often is abnormal in individuals who do not have coronary heart disease (CHD), but who have risk factors. Moreover, the development of cardiovascular complications in individuals who have IR depends not only on the severity of IR, but also on their ability to compensate for these defects and the presence of associated comorbidities [10].

Several large epidemiologic studies identified hyperinsulinemia as an independent cardiovascular risk factor or CHD precursor: the Busselton Study in Australia [13], the Helsinki Policeman Study in Finland [14], the Paris Prospective Study in France [15], and the San Antonio Heart Study in the United States [16]. Moreover, investigators in the Bruneck Study [17], performed in Italy, observed a U-shaped curved that linked fasting plasma insulin, 2 hours post-OGTT plasma insulin with CHD. This relationship persisted after adjustment for other cardiovascular risk factors, although lost some statistical power. Finally, the Quebec Cardiovascular Study unequivocally demonstrated the fasting insulin is an independent cardiovascular risk factor after adjustment for dyslipidemia and other cardiovascular variables; nevertheless, other studies showed contradictory results [18].

IR promotes the development of atherosclerosis through different mechanisms: through changes in the lipid profile (ie, atherogenic dyslipidemia), by increasing levels of plasminogen activator inhibitor-1 and fibrinogen, by increasing vascular tone and reactivity, and by inducing endothelial dysfunction [18].

Primary hyperparathyroidism as a cardiovascular risk factor

PHPT is susceptible to induce an increase in the incidence and prevalence of cardiovascular disease, either by hypercalcemia itself or through the effects of parathormone. Nevertheless, there are insufficient studies to prove causality between PHPT and cardiovascular disease [19–21].

Scattered medical literature states an association between IR and PHPT. Moreover, the results are not reproducible, and the reversibility of the cardiovascular risk upon surgical correction of hypercalcemia (ie, after parathyroidectomy) remains to be proven [21]. On the contrary, the presence of PTH-secreting adenomas is an additional cardiovascular risk factor in the natural course of CHD.

Several studies have reported a tendency toward vascular calcification in carotid intima media thickness evaluated with supra-aortic ultrasounds in PHPT. The increased carotid intima media thickness does not resolve after surgical correction of hypercalcemia [22,23].

The incidence of peri-operative cardiovascular complications is increased significantly in patients who have PHPT in the United States and Europe. Additionally, prospective studies confirmed true increases in the incidence and prevalence of cardiovascular events in these patients [21,23–26]. Conversely, no study has assessed the hypothetical link between IR and bone remodeling markers before and after surgical correction of PHPT.

The prevalence of HTN is increased in patients who have PHPT, and, occasionally, it persists after correction of hypercalcemia [27]. Conversely, fully reversible heart failure (with systolic and diastolic dysfunction) is reported in association with PHPT [28].

The relationship between PHPT and disturbances in lipid profiles (low high-density lipoprotein cholesterol levels, high triglyceride levels, and small, dense low-density lipoprotein cholesterol particles) improves upon surgical cure of PHPT [26]. The physiopathologic pathway that links hyperparathyroidism and atherogenic dyslipidemia has not been elucidated.

A few studies have reported the coincidence between the onset of T2DM and PHPT [29,30]. Indeed, the coexistence of T2DM in patients who have PHPT is an accepted criterion for urgent parathyroidectomy [31].

PHPT seems to coexist with a significant increase in glucose intolerance and T2DM prevalence. There seems to be peripheral and hepatic IR. The degree of IR correlates directly with iPTH levels [32–35]. PHPT, glucose intolerance, and IR coexist, and probable act synergistically in the natural course of cardiovascular disease [34]. Some investigators reported that IR disappeared after successful parathyroidectomy [34], and its effects on cardiovascular lesions are only transient.

The first studies that addressed the relationship between IR and PHPT appeared almost 3 decades ago [35,36], and, paradoxically, were mostly forgotten until the increase in prevalence of the IR syndrome.

IR is considered by most experts to be an epidemic condition that dramatically increases the risk for developing T2DM, CHD, stroke, and various cancers; it is estimated to affect at least one in three adults in the United States [1].

The radial artery flux and its intima media thickness were reported to be directly correlated with parathormone levels, which confirmed previous findings [37,38] on hyperparathyroidism and cardiovascular disease. Moreover, studies demonstrated the existence of endothelial dysfunction associated with PHPT and iPTH levels [38].

The availability of a full array of new markers of endothelial dysfunction—the earliest stage of atherosclerosis—and the likelihood of direct/

indirect relationships with hyperparathyroidism contribute to an increased understanding of the natural history of cardiovascular disease. These new findings will be integrated into the network of classic cardiovascular risk factors and the hypothetical relationship with genetic alterations.

Acknowledgments

The study was supported by (1) Fondo de Investigación Sanitaria (FIS) SPAIN, Grant # 01/0846 and Spanish Network CO3/08: Instituto Carlos III. Metabolism and nutrition illness and (2) Fondo de Investigación Sanitaria (FIS) SPAIN, grant number 01/0846. Spanish Network CO3/08: Instituto Carlos III. Metabolism and nutrition illness.

Further readings

Chiu KC, Chuang LM, Lee NP, et al. Insulin sensitivity is inversely correlated with plasma intact parathyroid hormone level. Metabolism 2000;49(11):1501–5.

Garcia de la Torre N, Wass JA, Turner HE. Parathyroid adenomas and cardiovascular risk. Endocr Relat Cancer 2003;10(2):309–22.

McCarty MF, Thomas CA. PTH excess may promote weight gain by impeding catecholamine-induced lipolysis-implications for the impact of calcium, vitamin D, and alcohol on body weight. Med Hypotheses 2003;61(5–6):535–42.

Piovesan A, Molineri N, Casasso F, et al. Left ventricular hypertrophy in primary hyperparathyroidism. Effects of successful parathyroidectomy. Clin Endocrinol (Oxf) 1999;50(3):321–8.

References

[1] American Diabetes Association. Consensus Development Conference on Insulin Resistance. Diabetes Care 1997;21(2):310–4.

[2] Ferranini E, Andrea M. How to measure insulin sensitivity. J Hypertens 1998;16:895–906.

[3] Albareda M, Rodriguez Espinosa J, Murugo M, et al. Assessment of insulin sensitivity and beta-cell function from measurement in the fasting state and during an oral glucose tolerance test. Diabetologia 1998;43:1507–11.

[4] Zierath JR, Krook A, Wallberg-Henriksson H. Insulin action and insulin resistance in human skeletal muscle. Diabetologia 2000;43:821–35.

[5] DeFronzo RA, Obin JD, Andres R. Glucose clamp technique: a method for quantifying insulin secretion and resistance. Am J Physiol 1979;237:E214–23.

[6] Stumvoll M, Mitrakou A, Pimenta W, et al. Use the oral glucose tolerance test to assess insulin release and insulin sensitivity. Diabetes Care 2000;23:295–301.

[7] Clark PMS, Hales CN. How to measure plasma insulin. Diabetes Metab Rev 1994;10:79–90.

[8] Matthews DR, Hosker JP, Rudenski AS, et al. Homeostasis model assessment: insulin resistance and beta-cell function from fasting plasma glucose and insulin concentrations in man. Diabetologia 1985;28:412–9.

[9] Robbins DC, Andersen L, Bowsher R, et al. Report of the American Diabetes Association's Task Force on Standardization of the Insulin Assay. Diabetes 1996;45:242–56.

[10] Proceedings of worldwide insulin resistance. Diabetes Obes Metab 1999;1(Suppl 1):1–50.

[11] Egan BM, Greene EL, Goodfriend TL. Insulin resistance and cardiovascular disease. Am J Hypertens 2001;14:116S–25S.

[12] Zavaroni I, Bonora E, Pagliara M, et al. Risk factors for coronary artery disease in healthy persons with hyperinsulinemia and normal glucose tolerance. N Engl J Med 1989;320:702–6.

[13] Welborn TA, Wearne K. Coronary heart disease incidence and cardiovascular mortality in Busselton with reference to glucose and insulin concentrations. Diabetes Care 1979;2:154–60.

[14] Pyorala M, Miettinen H, Laakso M, et al. Hyperinsulinemia predicts coronary heart disease risk in healthy middle-aged men: the 22-year follow-up results of the Helsinki Policemen Study. Circulation 1998;98(5):398–404.

[15] Ducimetiere P, Eschwege E, Papoz L, et al. Relationship of plasma insulin levels to the incidence of myocardial infarction and coronary heart disease mortality in a middle-aged population. Diabetologia 1980;19(3):205–10.

[16] Ferrannini E, Haffner SM, Mitchell BD, et al. Hyperinsulinaemia: the key feature of a cardiovascular and metabolic syndrome. Diabetologia 1991;34(6):416–22.

[17] Bonora E, Willeit J, Kiechl S, et al. U-shaped and J-shaped relationships between serum insulin and coronary heart disease in the general population. The Bruneck Study. Diabetes Care 1998;21(2):221–30.

[18] Ruige JB, Assendelft WJ, Dekker JM, et al. Insulin and risk of cardiovascular disease: a meta-analysis. Circulation 1998;97(10):996–1001.

[19] Melton LJ III. The epidemiology of primary hyperparathyroidism in North America. J Bone Miner Res 2002;17(Suppl 2):N12–7.

[20] Ogard CG, Engholm G, Almdal TP, et al. Increased mortality in patients hospitalized with primary hyperparathyroidism during the period 1977–1993 in Denmark. World J Surg 2004;28(1):108–11.

[21] Vestergaard P, Mosekilde L. Cohort study on effects of parathyroid surgery on multiple outcomes in primary hyperparathyroidism. BMJ 2003;327(7414):530–4.

[22] Fallo F, Camporese G, Capitelli E, et al. Ultrasound evaluation of carotid artery in primary hyperparathyroidism. J Clin Endocrinol Metab 2003;88(5):2096–9.

[23] Nuzzo V, Tauchmanova L, Fonderico F, et al. Increased intima-media thickness of the carotid artery wall, normal blood pressure profile and normal left ventricular mass in subjects with primary hyperparathyroidism. Eur J Endocrinol 2002;147(4):453–9.

[24] Vestergaard P, Mollerup CL, Frokjaer VG, et al. Cardiovascular events before and after surgery for primary hyperparathyroidism. World J Surg 2003;27(2):216–22.

[25] Nilsson IL, Yin L, Lundgren E, et al. Clinical presentation of primary hyperparathyroidism in Europe–nationwide cohort analysis on mortality from nonmalignant causes. J Bone Miner Res 2002;17(Suppl 2):N68–74.

[26] Hedback GM, Oden AS. Cardiovascular disease, hypertension and renal function in primary hyperparathyroidism. J Intern Med 2002;251(6):476–83.

[27] Hagstrom E, Lundgren E, Lithell H, et al. Normalized dyslipidaemia after parathyroidectomy in mild primary hyperparathyroidism: population-based study over five years. Clin Endocrinol (Oxf) 2002;56(2):253–60.

[28] Nilsson IL, Aberg J, Rastad J, et al. Left ventricular systolic and diastolic function and exercise testing in primary hyperparathyroidism-effects of parathyroidectomy. Surgery 2000;128(6):895–902.

[29] Procopio M, Magro G, Cesario F, et al. The oral glucose tolerance test reveals a high frequency of both impaired glucose tolerance and undiagnosed type 2 diabetes mellitus in primary hyperparathyroidism. Diabet Med 2002;19(11):958–61.

[30] Taylor WH, Khaleeli AA. Coincident diabetes mellitus and primary hyperparathyroidism. Diabetes Metab Res Rev 2001;17(3):175–80.

[31] Richards ML, Thompson NW. Diabetes mellitus with hyperparathyroidism: another indication for parathyroidectomy? Surgery 1999;126(6):1160–6.

[32] Kumar S, Olukoga AO, Gordon C, et al. Impaired glucose tolerance and insulin insensitivity in primary hyperparathyroidism. Clin Endocrinol (Oxf) 1994;40(1):47–53.

[33] Kautzky-Willer A, Pacini G, Niederle B, et al. Insulin secretion, insulin sensitivity and hepatic insulin extraction in primary hyperparathyroidism before and after surgery. Clin Endocrinol (Oxf) 1992;37(2):147–55.

[34] Prager R, Schernthaner G, Niederle B, et al. Evaluation of glucose tolerance, insulin secretion, and insulin action in patients with primary hyperparathyroidism before and after surgery. Calcif Tissue Int 1990;46(1):1–4.

[35] Prager R, Kovarik J, Schernthaner G, et al. Peripheral insulin resistance in primary hyperparathyroidism. Metabolism 1983;32(8):800–5.

[36] Ginsberg H, Olefsky JM, Reaven GM. Evaluation of insulin resistance in patients with primary hyperparathyroidism. Proc Soc Exp Biol Med 1975;148(3):942–5.

[37] Kosch M, Hausberg M, Vormbrock K, et al. Studies on flow-mediated vasodilation and intima-media thickness of the brachial artery in patients with primary hyperparathyroidism. Am J Hypertens 2000;13(7):759–64.

[38] Nilsson IL, Aberg J, Rastad J, et al. Endothelial vasodilatory dysfunction in primary hyperparathyroidism is reversed after parathyroidectomy. Surgery 1999;126(6):1049–55.

ELSEVIER
SAUNDERS

NURSING
CLINICS
OF NORTH AMERICA

Nurs Clin N Am 42 (2007) 87–99

Hypogonadal Hypogonadism and Osteoporosis in Men

June Hart Romeo, PhD, NP-C[a],*,
Juan Ybarra, MD, PhD, FACE[b]

[a]MedCentral College of Nursing, 335 Glessner Avenue Mansfield, Ohio 44903, USA
[b]Servicio de Endocrinología y Nutrición, Hospital de Sant Pau, Barcelona, Spain

In recent years, osteoporosis in men has become increasingly recognized as an important clinical and public health problem. Many similarities exist in various aspects of osteoporosis in men and women, but this article focuses on the sex difference, bone biology, epidemiology, and consequences of fractures. Although maintenance of bone integrity depends on the action of sex hormones in both sexes, menopause is a much more obvious indicator of estrogen deficiency than is the subtle decrease of testosterone in aging men. This often leads to delay and neglect of diagnosis. The need to identify and screen men at particular risk for osteoporosis, as when hypogonadism is induced for treatment of prostate cancer, has become important. Secondary causes of osteoporosis are more prominent in men, so a thorough evaluation of these factors is important.

The appropriate use of testosterone for prevention and treatment of osteoporosis is reviewed, as well as the potential value of future selective androgen receptor modulators. The roles of bisphosphonates and teriparatide also are discussed.

Epidemiology and risk of fracture

Although not as common as in women, osteoporosis in men is not rare [1]. Using the World Health Organization guidelines for diagnosing osteoporosis, 1 to 2 million men in the United States have osteoporosis, and another 8 to 13 million have osteopenia [2]. Thirteen percent of men older than 50 years of age will have an osteoporotic fracture later in life [3]. Approximately 30% of all hip fractures occur in men [4]. The morbidity and

* Corresponding author.
E-mail address: jromeo@medcentral.edu (J.H. Romeo).

0029-6465/07/$ - see front matter © 2007 Elsevier Inc. All rights reserved.
doi:10.1016/j.cnur.2006.11.004   *nursing.theclinics.com*

mortality associated with hip and vertebral fractures seem to be higher in men [5]. Fifty percent of men need institutionalized care after a hip fracture, compared with just 30% of women, and men are twice as likely to die in the hospital following a hip fracture [6]. The 1-year mortality after hip fracture is 31% in men, compared with 17% in women [7]. Hip fractures tend to occur about 10 years later in men than women [8,9]. The higher mortality may be the result of more comorbid conditions at any specific age and the shorter life expectancy in men at time of fracture [10].

Bone biology in male patients

Recent consensus statements on osteoporosis in men suggest that measurement of bone mineral density (BMD) at the spine and hip predicts fracture risk in a way comparable to that in women [10]. Despite similarities, there are important differences in the development of the skeletons of male and female patients to be considered. Differences in sex-related fracture rates often have been attributed to a higher BMD in men [11]. At any age, a lower proportion of men sustain fractures, because fewer men have the structural determinants of bone strength below a critical level at which loads exceed bone strength [12]. Some significant differences in bone structure between the sexes start at puberty. Before puberty in both sexes, the length and width of bone increase progressively [11]. The onset of puberty is later in boys, so longitudinal growth, particularly at the appendicular skeleton, continues longer and accounts for the increased height in boys at skeletal maturity [10]. Men achieve greater peak bone mass—by about 8% to 10% when areal density is measured—and this likely confers a mechanical advantage, although peak volumetric density differs little between the sexes [2]. Peak vertebral bone density in terms of trabecular number and thickness is equal in young men and women. Bone width is greater in men, however, which lead to a greater peak vertebral size and greater bone strength [5]. Hypothetically, their larger and stronger muscles put greater stress on bone, which would result in increased bone formation. Genetics also may play a role, because sex-specific genes that contribute to peak BMD have been identified [13]. In addition to larger skeletons at peak, men have less architectural disruption, and skeletons that adapt better to aging in terms of periosteal apposition [12]. Sex differences in BMD tend to be skeletal site–dependent; appendicular skeletal sites with a larger proportion of cortical bone have the greatest sex disparity [11].

Role of sex hormones in relation to bone loss

Generally, bone mass is maintained well in men, with slow but perceptible changes over time [2]. Men lose less bone mass than women do during the middle years because there is no menopause equivalent [2]. Aging is associated with a decline in total serum testosterone and a greater decrease in free testosterone, in part because of an increase in sex hormone–binding globulin. Some aging men have a reduced production of testosterone with a decreased bone mass and may or may not have symptoms of hypogonadism.

Good evidence shows the relation between low testosterone and osteoporosis. Hypogonadism is more common in men with fragility fractures than in age-matched controls [10]. Long-standing testosterone deficiency is typical of approximately 30% of men who present with spinal osteoporosis [14]. Testosterone is converted to estrogen in adipose tissue and is important for the bones of men as well as women. Gradual reductions in estradiol (E2), in particular in the bioavailable form, occur during aging as with testosterone [15]. A reduction in estrogen levels is related more closely to reduced bone mass and increased bone turnover than declining androgen levels [2,16,17]. Quantitative CT has been used at peripheral and central sites to study the effects of bioavailable E2 and testosterone on trabecular and cortical bone in men with age-associated bone changes [18]. Bioavailable E2 was the best predictor of volumetric BMD and some geometric variables [18]. Although androgens and estrogens contribute to the maintenance of skeletal health in men, the precise role of each sex steroid remains to be defined.

Effect of androgen replacement on bone

Androgens have skeletal actions that are clearly different from those of estrogens [19]. One of these actions is to increase periosteal bone formation, which increases bone size and plays an important role in decreasing fracture risk [19]. Recent findings suggest, however, that estrogens are essential during puberty for the process of periosteal bone expansion that is associated with the male bone phenotype [20].

Although long-term testosterone replacement may increase BMD of the spine by as much as 25%, this generally occurs during the first 2 years. There seems to be an inverse relation between the pretreatment serum testosterone and the response to treatment, so that the maximum effect occurs when the testosterone level is very low and there is little change when basal testosterone is normal [21–23]. Physiologic amounts of androgen given to older men do not improve bone density convincingly [24]. Current guidelines from the American Association of Clinical Endocrinologists state that men with a total testosterone level of less than 200 ng/dL and who have symptomatic hypogonadism are potential candidates for therapy. To emphasize, testosterone is not recommended solely for improving BMD and does not have a role in preventing or treating osteoporosis in eugonadal men. It is customary to replace with testosterone (gel) when testosterone deficiency is clinically apparent and less than 200 ng/dL in two morning blood samples. Although it is possible that elderly men whose testosterone levels are not quite as low may benefit from treatment, until the safety and efficacy of treating this group are established, the prudent course is to limit treatment to the more severely hypogonadal because they are more likely to benefit [25].

An important recent study reported that intramuscular testosterone, given for 26 months to 50 elderly hypogonadal men, caused a 9% to 10% increase in BMD at the lumbar spine and a 2% to 3% increase at the hip compared with placebo [26]. The impressive BMD changes noted in this study likely were a result of the higher dose of testosterone used compared with other studies; unfortunately, this also was associated with a higher frequency of adverse effects [27]. The addition of finasteride to testosterone replacement did not diminish the increases seen in BMD, and a decrease was noted in prostate growth and in the increase of prostate-specific antigen with this dual treatment, compared with testosterone alone or placebo [26]. Improvement in the hip is not supported by other studies [21]. The lesser effect on hip, compared with spine, probably relates to the greater effect of sex steroids on trabecular bone than cortical bone. This is analogous to the lesser increase in BMD at the hip than spine with estrogen treatment of women after menopause [22].

The effect of testosterone on the bone in hypogonadal men occurs regardless of age [28]. Testosterone may have a lesser effect in patients who have secondary hypogonadism [29]. In secondary hypogonadism, other deficiencies, such as growth hormone, may play a role in the osteoporosis [22].

Prevention of osteoporosis and fractures

People of all ages should be aware of how to optimize their bone health and prevent future fractures. Although certain biologic and environmental factors lend more protection against fractures to men (Box 1), preventive

---

Box 1. Reasons why men are less likely than women to develop osteoporosis and fragility fractures

More physically active throughout life, especially when young
Tend to drink more milk during childhood and adolescence
Greater areal density and cross-sectional area of bone
No pregnancy or nursing[a]
Less likely to have eating disorders, such as anorexia nervosa
No menopause equivalent with abrupt lowering of sex hormone levels

---

[a] Problematic when dietary deficiencies are insufficient to support the needs of the fetus or infant as maternal bone resorption is increased. *From* U.S. Department of Health and Human Services. The 2004 Surgeon General's Report on Bone Health and Osteoporosis: What It Means To You. U.S. Department of Health and Human Services, Office of the Surgeon General, 2004.

measures, such as not abusing alcohol, are important. Smoking of tobacco significantly increases the risk for fracture in older men [30].

According to a recent cross-sectional study, higher consumption of dairy foods was associated with increased hip BMD in older men [31]. Medications that are known to potentiate bone loss, such as anticonvulsants, anticoagulants, and excessive steroids, should be avoided or minimized, and the need for androgen replacement therapy should be considered when hypogonadism is suspected. Regular weight-bearing exercise throughout life is important.

Male athletes older than 60 years who retire from sports lose exercise-induced BMD benefits, but have fewer fractures than do matched controls [32]. Moderate weight loss may be detrimental to bones, because older men who experience weight loss have increased rates of bone loss at the hip, even among overweight and obese men who undergo voluntary weight reductions [33].

Hypovitaminosis D is a subject of increasing interest and importance. Many recent publications document the worldwide prevalence of vitamin D deficiency in all populations. The classic action of vitamin D in preventing rickets, osteomalacia, and hypocalcemia is well known. Recently, more subtle actions of vitamin D have been recognized, including its role in preventing osteoporosis and the maintenance of muscle strength and function [34]. Evidence is evolving for a role of vitamin D in the prevention of certain cancers and autoimmune diseases [35].

The Surgeon General's report on osteoporosis recommends 400 to 600 IU/d on the basis of information available in 1997. In a recent study, a vitamin D intake of 400 IU/d was not sufficient for fracture prevention, whereas 700 to 800 IU/d reduced the risk for hip and other nonvertebral fractures in ambulatory or institutionalized elderly persons [36]. The minimum serum level of 25-hydroxyvitamin D needed for optimal bone health has been discussed considerably [37,38].

Most vitamin D experts estimate that the mean minimal level of serum 25 hydroxyvitamin D needed for an optimal effect on fracture prevention is 30 ng/mL, and that the mean oral intake of cholecalciferol needed to reach this level is 1100 IU/d [39]. These data confirm that hypovitaminosis D is much more common than previously believed, and that it is likely that vitamin D supplementation may prevent many fractures, particularly in the elderly. Ultraviolet irradiation of the skin from exposure to sunlight is a potentially important, but generally unreliable, source of vitamin D. An adequate amount of vitamin D is difficult to obtain from food, so vitamin D supplementation is usually needed.

The preservation of muscle strength and balance and the prevention of falls are important in reducing fracture risk. Most hip fractures are preceded by a fall, and important sex-specific differences have been noted [40]. Fall frequency is lower in elderly men than in elderly women; when women fall, they are more likely than men to land on the hip, and, thus, are at a higher risk for fracture.

A recent study showed that elderly men with a lower relative skeletal muscle mass have an impaired balance and an increased risk for falls [41]. Vitamin D deficiency also has been recognized to cause muscle weakness and correlate with falls [42]. Vitamin D supplementation of vitamin D–deficient elderly people improved muscle strength and functional ability and reduced falls and nonvertebral fractures [42]. Escalation of testosterone doses to older men may be particularly effective on muscle mass and strength [43]. The frequency of adverse effects makes long-term use unlikely, however. The data do provide evidence that some age-related changes in body composition and muscle strength are reversible [43].

No therapeutic agents are approved by the US Food and Drug Administration (FDA) for prevention of osteoporosis in men. Oral alendronate, risedronate, and intravenous pamidronate are used for this indication, however, especially when the onset of a medical condition is acute and progressive osteoporosis is expected, as occurs in patients who receive androgen deprivation therapy or those who are immobilized [44–46]. The doses and contraindications are the same as for prevention of osteoporosis in women.

Screening

Osteoporosis in men commonly presents with a vertebral or hip fracture, whereas in women it is diagnosed more often by routine BMD screening [47]. As the prevalence of osteoporosis in men is recognized more widely, the goal is earlier diagnosis and treatment of men at high fracture risk. Box 2 lists some factors in male patients that indicate a greater chance of osteoporosis and warrant further evaluation. Most endocrinologists advocate the incorporation of diabetic educators to assist in screening patients who have diabetes for osteoporosis, because there has been increasing evidence that people who have type 1 or type 2 diabetes are at an increased risk for fragility fracture [48]. Patients who have type 2 diabetes tend to

---

Box 2. Indications for bone mineral density testing in men

Current or past fragility fracture
Family history of osteoporosis
Lack of calcium, vitamin D intake
Loss of more than 1.5 inches in height
Vertebral deformity or osteopenia seen on radiograph
Chronic use of corticosteroids
Presence of disease known to cause bone loss
All men older than 70 years of age

fracture with a normal BMD [49]. This may be a result of poor quality of bone, an increased risk for falling, or both.

Hip fracture rates can be predicted accurately from age and BMD in men and women [50]. In women, a larger proportion of hip fractures occur at a T-score less than −2.5 than in men using the same absolute BMD threshold; however, using a male-specific T-score largely solves this diagnostic problem [51]. The current International Society of Clinical Densitometry (ISCD) guidelines on the use of T-scores in men for diagnosing osteoporosis are listed in Table 1 [52].

In men and women, age-related bone loss begins at about 50 years of age; however, acute hypogonadism at any age, such as that resulting from orchiectomy or gonadotropin-releasing hormone, accelerates bone loss [47,53,54]. These patients need aggressive screening and treatment for bone loss. The risk for osteoporotic fractures is increased in this population; contributing factors include depleted bone density and an increased tendency to fall because of muscle weakness–impaired balance [55–57].

A BMD measurement should be taken when beginning androgen-deprivation therapy; it should be repeated in 1 year and at appropriate intervals thereafter [55]. Bone markers also may provide an early detection of BMD loss during androgen-deprivation therapy [58]. Traumatic brain injury is increasingly common in young men and often causes anterior pituitary dysfunction, including hypogonadism [59].

Treatment of osteoporosis in men

Before initiating therapy of established osteoporosis (see Table 1) [60], secondary causes should be considered and addressed if possible, along with other lifestyle factors (see Prevention of Osteoporosis and Fractures). Nutritional deficiencies, especially calcium, should be corrected. All patients who are referred for treatment of osteoporosis should have their vitamin D status assessed by measuring serum 25 hydroxyvitamin D levels. Values of 30 ng/mL and greater are considered normal (optimal) [39]. For values less than 20 ng/mL, 50,000 IU ergocalciferol (Drisdol) is prescribed weekly for 8 weeks; when serum levels normalize, patients are advised to take 1000

Table 1
Use of T-scores in the diagnosis of osteoporosis in men based on age and associated risk factors

Population (men only)	Diagnosis of osteoporosis
Age ≥65 y	T-scores using World Health Organization criteria
Age ≥50 y but <65 y	Need both T-score at or below −2.5 and other risk factors for fracture
Age <50 y	Should not be made on basis of T-score alone

Men at any age with a fragility fracture may be diagnosed with osteoporosis, even without a low bone mineral density.

to 1200 IU cholecalciferol daily from food and dietary supplements. This is the maintenance amount that is advised for all patients, except those who have malabsorption or liver or kidney problems. Although cholecalciferol is the preferred form of vitamin D, 50,000-IU preparations are not available in the United States [61].

Another problem is the variability between laboratories in the measurement of vitamin D [62].

The agents that are used to treat men who have established osteoporosis are oral bisphosphonates (alendronate and risedronate), teriparatide, and, on occasion, intravenous pamidronate. Exclusion criteria and dosage of these agents are the same as for women. The evidence of efficacy used in treating osteoporosis in men is much less than for women, and sometimes is based on results of clinical trials in women. Alendronate is FDA-approved for decreasing the risk for vertebral fractures and increasing BMD of the hip. In six studies since 2000 [63–68], alendronate increased BMD of vertebrae and hip, including in patients who had hypogonadism [63,68]. Three papers reported prevention of vertebral fractures [65,67,68]. None reported a decreased risk for hip fractures. Bone turnover markers were decreased in two studies [64,67]. Alendronate taken weekly is now available in combination with 2800 IU of cholecalciferol. Risedronate is not FDA-approved for treatment of male osteoporosis (with the exception of glucocorticoid-induced osteoporosis). Ringe and colleagues [69] reported that risedronate increased vertebral and hip BMD and prevented vertebral fractures.

Teriparatide is FDA-approved for preventing vertebral fractures and increasing BMD of the hip in men. As in women, teriparatide should be used only in patients with serious risk for fracture and has all the exclusion criteria as for women.

Three studies since 2000 [70–72] demonstrated an increase of BMD in spine and hip with teriparatide, but only Kaufman and colleagues [70] demonstrated a decrease in vertebral fractures. None reported a decreased risk for hip fractures. Two papers reported an increase in bone turnover markers [71,72]. Alendronate seems to impair the ability of teriparatide to increase vertebral and hip BMD [73]. In contrast, oral bisphosphonates can help to maintain the increases in BMD that are obtained from treatment with teriparatide [70]. The use of testosterone is appropriate for management of hypogonadal symptoms, but the treatment of osteoporosis in men with low testosterone should be with a bisphosphonate or teriparatide. Pamidronate, generally 60 mg intravenously over a period of 3 hours every 3 months, is not FDA-approved for the treatment of osteoporosis; however, it is used sometimes when patients cannot tolerate or have failed to respond to treatment with the first three agents. Prevention of falls and use of hip protectors are important to reduce the incidence of hip fractures, especially in the frail elderly [47]. Orwoll [16] wrote a more detailed discussion on the treatment of osteoporosis in men. The undertreatment of patients who have osteoporosis, men included, has become a major public health problem and a major reason for the publication for the 2004 Surgeon General's Report on Bone Health and Osteoporosis.

Some patients do not respond to treatment with the aforementioned therapeutic agents. In these particular patients, it seems appropriate to measure 24-hour urine calcium (and creatinine). In the presence of normal serum calcium, urine calcium may be low or even undetectable. This reflects calcium malabsorption and even may occur in asymptomatic patients with low or normal levels of 25-hydroxyvitamin D. Appropriate history and laboratory tests often reveal the presence of celiac or Crohn's disease. These patients are resistant to the action of vitamin D and respond to treatment with large doses of vitamin D, along with gluten restriction in patients who have celiac disease [74].

Potential treatment options

At least two antiresorptive treatments for osteoporosis are in late-phase testing. One is zoledronic acid, a bisphosphonate already marketed for several cancer-related conditions. As a yearly 15-minute infusion, it should simplify treatment and assure compliance. The second is an inhibitor of the receptor activator of nuclear factor-κB ligand inhibitor made by Amgen (Thousand Oaks, CA) [75]. Two anabolic agents being tested are parathyroid hormone (PTH) 1-84 and PTHrp. Several androgen-receptor modulators are in various phases of development and would be expected to stimulate desired organs (bone, muscle) without stimulating the prostate [76].

Assessment of response to treatment

ISCD guidelines state that serial BMD testing can be used to monitor response to therapy by finding an increase or stability of bone density. Sequential bone densities should be performed on the same machine. The interval between BMD testing is generally 1 to 2 years, according to each patient's clinical status. Although a low BMD is an important risk factor for osteoporotic fractures, other determinants of bone strength are not measurable by BMD [77]. High bone turnover may be associated with an increased risk for osteoporotic fracture in elderly men (as in women) independent of BMD, and perhaps bone turnover markers used in combination with BMD measurements could improve fracture risk prediction. The increase in bone-specific alkaline phosphatase may predict the efficacy of teriparatide in preventing fractures [78]. Although useful in population studies, lack of precision limits the value of following bone turnover markers in individual, treated patients, and it is not our general approach at this time [79].

Beyond BMD testing, some newer, noninvasive techniques to assess resistance to fracture are being investigated, but are not clinically available. These include three-dimensional magnetic resonance microimaging, micro-computed tomography, and direct image analysis [80].

Summary

Osteoporosis in men is becoming recognized as an important health problem. The diagnosis and treatment of at-risk individuals remain underappreciated, however. Important sex-specific differences exist in bone physiology and geometry, fracture epidemiology, bone gonadal hormone response, and mortality after hip fracture [40].

One of the main differences between men and women in evaluating the cause of osteoporosis is the clarity of menopause and the subtlety of androgen deficiency. The risk for osteoporosis increases as a consequence of declining testosterone levels, and although bone density can be improved with testosterone replacement therapy, lack of fracture reduction data and safety concerns are limiting issues. The effect of androgen therapy is less clear in men with normal gonadal function, who represent most men who have osteoporosis [60].

The role of estrogen in conjunction with androgens in maintaining the male skeleton has been recognized and may have future implications in treatment.

The oral bisphosphonates and teriparatide are the primary means of treating male osteoporosis. The importance of adequate calcium and vitamin D intake, weight-bearing exercise, and avoidance of substances (eg, tobacco) that reduce bone density should be emphasized for prevention and during treatment. We look forward to improvements in diagnosing and monitoring treatment by using new radiologic techniques that would better assess bone quality and improve standardized assays for bone turnover markers and vitamin D. Emerging treatment options hold promise for our patients in the future.

References

[1] Kanis JA, Johnell O, Oden A, et al. Epidemiology of osteoporosis and fracture in men. Calcif Tissue Int 2004;75:90–9.

[2] Bilezikian JP. Commentary: osteoporosis in men. J Clin Endocrinol Metab 1999;84:3431–4.

[3] Melton LJ III, Chrischilles EA, Cooper C, et al. How many women have osteoporosis? J Bone Miner Res 1992;7:1005–10.

[4] Cooper C, Melton LJ III. Epidemiology of osteoporosis. Trends Endocrinol Metab 1992;3: 224–9.

[5] Seeman E. During aging, men lose less bone than women because they gain more periosteal bone, not because they resorb less endosteal bone. Calcif Tissue Int 2001;69:205–8.

[6] Diamond TH, Thornley SW, Sekel R, et al. Hip fracture in elderly men: prognostic factors and outcomes. Med J Aust 1997;167:412–5.

[7] Forsen L, Sogaard AJ, Meyer HE, et al. Survival after hip fracture: short and long-term excess mortality according to age and gender. Osteoporos Int 1999;10:73–8.

[8] Farmer ME, White LR, Brody JA, et al. Race and sex difference in hip fracture incidence. Am J Public Health 1984;74:1374–80.

[9] Center JR, Nguyen TV, Schneider D, et al. Mortality after all types of osteoporotic fractures in men and women: an observational study. Lancet 1999;353:878–82.

[10] Seeman E, Bianchi G, Adami S, et al. Osteoporosis in men — consensus is premature. Calcif Tissue Int 2004;75:120–2.

[11] Nieves JW, Formica C, Ruffing J, et al. Males have larger skeletal size and bone mass than females, despite comparable body size. J Bone Miner Res 2005;20:529–35.

[12] Seeman E. The growth and age-related origins of bone fragility in men. Calcif Tissue Int 2004;75:100–9.

[13] Peacock M, Koller DL, Fishburn T, et al. Sex-specific and non-sex-specific quantitative trait loci contribute to normal variation in bone mineral density in men. J Clin Endocrinol Metab 2005;90:3060–6.

[14] Jackson JA, Kleerekoper M, Parfitt AM, et al. Frame B: bone histomorphometry in hypogonadal and eugonadal men with spinal osteoporosis. J Clin Endocrinol Metab 1987;65: 53–8.

[15] Khosla S, Melton LJ III, Riggs BL. Estrogens and bone health in men. Calcif Tissue Int 2001; 69:189–92.

[16] Orwoll ES. Treatment of osteoporosis in men. Calcif Tissue Int 2004;75:114–9.

[17] Szulc P, Munoz F, Claustrat B, et al. Bioavailable estradiol may be an important determinant of osteoporosis in men: the MINOS study. J Clin Endocrinol Metab 2001;86:192–9.

[18] Khosla S, Melton LJ III, Robb RA, et al. Relationship of volumetric BMD and structural parameters at different skeletal sites to sex steroid levels in men. J Bone Miner Res 2005; 20:730–40.

[19] Orwoll ES. Androgens: basic biology and clinical implication. Calcif Tissue Int 2001;69: 185–8.

[20] Boullion R, Bex M, Vanderschueren D, et al. Estrogens are essential for male pubertal periosteal bone expansion. J Clin Endocrinol Metab 2004;89:6025–9.

[21] Francis RM. Androgen replacement in aging men. Calcif Tissue Int 2001;69:235–8.

[22] Snyder PJ, Peachey H, Hannoush P, et al. Effect of testosterone treatment on bone mineral density in men over 65 years of age. J Clin Endocrinol Metab 1999;84:1966–72.

[23] Snyder PJ. Effects of age on testicular function and consequences of testosterone treatment. J Clin Endocrinol Metab 2001;86:2369–72.

[24] Liu PY, Swerdloff RS, Veldhuis JD. The rationale, efficacy and safety of androgen therapy in older men: future research and current practice recommendations. J Clin Endocrinol Metab 2004;89:4789–96.

[25] Snyder PJ. Hypogonadism in elderly men — what to do until the evidence comes. N Engl J Med 2004;350:440–2.

[26] Amory JK, Watts NB, Easley KA, et al. Exogenous testosterone or testosterona with finasteride increases bone mineral density in older men with low serum testosterone. J Clin Endocrinol Metab 2004;89:503–10.

[27] Barrett-Conner E, Bhasin S. Time for (more research on) testosterone [editorial]. J Clin Endocrinol Metab 2004;89:501–2.

[28] Behre HM, Kliesch S, Leifke E, et al. Long-term effect of testosterone therapy on bone mineral density in hypogonadal men. J Clin Endocrinol Metab 1997;82:2386–90.

[29] Schubert M, Bullmann C, Minnemann T, et al. Osteoporosis in male hypogonadism: responses to androgen substitution differ among men with primary and secondary hypogonadism. Horm Res 2003;60:21–8.

[30] Olofsson H, Byberg L, Mohsen R, et al. Smoking and the risk of fracture in older men. J Bone Miner Res 2005;20:1261–3.

[31] McCabe LD, Martin BR, McCabe GP, et al. Dairy intakes affect bone density in the elderly. Am J Clin Nutr 2004;80:1066–74.

[32] Nordstrom A, Karlsson C, Nyquist F, et al. Bone loss and fracture risk after reduced physical activity. J Bone Miner Res 2005;90:202–7.

[33] Ensrud KE, Fullman RL, Barrett-Connor E, et al. Voluntary weight reduction in older men increases hip bone loss: the Osteoporotic Fractures in Men Study. J Clin Endocrinol Metab 2005;90:1998–2004.

[34] Bischoff HA, Stahelin HB, Dick W, et al. Effects of vitamin D and calcium supplementation on falls, a randomized controlled trial. J Bone Miner Res 2003;18:343–51.

[35] Holick MF. Sunlight and vitamin D for bone health and prevention of autoimmune diseases, cancers, and cardiovascular disease. Am J Clin Nutr 2004;80(6 Suppl):1678S–88S.

[36] Bischoll-Ferrari HA, Willett WC, Wong JB, et al. Fracture prevention with vitamin D supplementation: a metaanalysis of randomized controlled trials. JAMA 2005;293:2257–64.

[37] Hollis BW, Wagner CL. Normal serum vitamin D levels. N Engl J Med 2005;352:515–6.

[38] Heaney RP. Functional indices of vitamin D status and ramifications of vitamin D deficiency. Am J Clin Nutr 2004;80(6 Suppl):1706S–9S.

[39] Dawson-Hughes B, Heaney RP, Holick MF, et al. Estimates of optimal vitamin D status. Osteoporos Int 2005;16:713–6.

[40] Boling EP. Gender and osteoporosis: similarities and sex-specific differences. J Gend Specif Med 2001;4:36–43.

[41] Szulc P, Beck TJ, Marchand F, et al. Low skeletal muscle mass is associated with poor structural parameters of bone and impaired balance in elderly men-the MINOS study. J Bone Miner Res 2005;20:721–9.

[42] Janessen HCJP, Samson MM, Verhaar HJJ. Vitamin D deficiency, muscle function, and falls in elderly people. Am J Clin Nutr 2002;75:611–5.

[43] Bhasin S, Woodhouse L, Casaburi R, et al. Older men are as responsive as young men to the anabolic effects of graded doses of testosterone on the skeletal muscle. J Clin Endocrinol Metab 2005;90:678–88.

[44] Smith MR, McGovern FJ, Zietman AL, et al. Pamidronate to prevent bone loss during androgen-deprivation therapy for prostate cancer. N Engl J Med 2001;345:948–55.

[45] van der Poest CE, van Engeland M, Ader H, et al. Alendronate in the prevention of bone loss after a fracture of the lower leg. J Bone Miner Res 2002;17:2247–55.

[46] Zehnder Y, Risi S, Knecht H, et al. Prevention of bone loss in paraplegics over 2 years with alendronate. J Bone Miner Res 2004;19(7):1067–74.

[47] Campion JM, Maricic MJ. Osteoporosis in men. Am Fam Physician 2003;67:1521–6.

[48] Kemmis K, Stuber D. Diabetes and osteoporotic fractures: the diabetes educator's role in screening, evaluating, treating, and referring. Todays Educ 2005;31:187–96.

[49] Schwartz AV, Sellmeyer DE, Strotmeyer ES, et al. Diabetes and bone loss at the hip in older black and white adults. J Bone Miner Res 2005;20:596–603.

[50] DeLaet CEDH, Van Hout BA, Burger H, et al. Hip fracture prediction in elderly men and women: validation in the Rotterdam Study. J Bone Miner Res 1998;13:1587–93.

[51] DeLaet CEDH, Van Der Klift M, Hofman A, et al. Osteoporosis in men and women: a story about bone mineral density thresholds and hip fracture risk. J Bone Miner Res 2002;17:2231–6.

[52] Leib ES, Lewiecki EM, Binkley N, et al. Official positions of the International Society for Clinical Densitometry. J Clin Densitom 2004;7:1–5.

[53] Mittan D, Lee S, Miller E, et al. Bone loss following hypogonadism in men with prostate cancer treated with GnRH analogs. J Clin Endocrinol Metab 2002;87:3656–61.

[54] Stoch SA, Parker RA, Chen L, et al. Bone loss in men with prostate cancer treated with gonadotropin-releasing hormone agonists. J Clin Endocrinol Metab 2001;86:2787–91.

[55] Daniell HW. Osteoporosis due to androgen deprivation therapy in men with prostate cancer. Urology 2001;58:101–7.

[56] Shahinian V, Kuo YF, Freeman JL, et al. Risk of fracture after androgen deprivation for prostate cancer. N Engl J Med 2005;352:154–64.

[57] Lopez AM, Pena MA, Hernandez R, et al. Fracture risk in patients with prostate cancer on androgen deprivation therapy. Osteoporos Int 2005;16:707–11.

[58] Nishiyama T, Ishizaki F, Anraku T, et al. The influence of androgen deprivation therapy on metabolism in patients with prostate cancer. J Clin Endocrinol Metab 2005;90:657–60.

[59] Agha A, Rogers B, Sherlock M, et al. Anterior pituitary dysfunction in survivors of traumatic brain injury. J Clin Endocrinol Metab 2004;89:4929–36.

[60] Olszynski WP, Davison KS, Adachi JD, et al. Osteoporosis in men: epidemiology, diagnosis, prevention, and treatment. Clin Ther 2004;26:15–28.

[61] Armas LA, Hollis BW, Heaney RP. Vitamin D2 is much less effective than vitamin D3 in humans. J Clin Endocrinol Metab 2004;89:5387–91.

[62] Binkley N, Drueger D, Cowgill CS, et al. Assay variation confounds the diagnosis of hypovitaminosis D: a call for standardization. J Clin Endocrinol Metab 2004;89:3152–7.

[63] Sawka AM, Thabane L, Papaioannou A, et al. A systematic review of the effect of alendronate on bone mineral density in men. J Clin Densitom 2005;8:7–13.

[64] Shimon I, Eshed V, Doolman R, et al. Alendronate for osteoporosis in men with androgen-repleted hypogonadism. Osteoporos Int 2005;16:1591–6.

[65] Ringe JD, Dorst A, Faber H, et al. Alendronate treatment of established primary osteoporosis in men: 3-year results of a prospective, comparative, two-arm study. Rheumatol Int 2004;24:110–3.

[66] Gonnelli S, Cepollaro C, Montagnani A, et al. Alendronate treatment in men with primary osteoporosis: a three-year longitudinal study. Calcif Tissue Int 2003;73:133–9.

[67] Ringe JD, Orwoll E, Daifotis A, et al. Treatment of male osteoporosis: recent advances with alendronate. Osteoporos Int 2002;13:195–9.

[68] Orwoll E, Ettinger M, Weiss S, et al. Alendronate for the treatment of osteoporosis in men. N Engl J Med 2000;343:604–10.

[69] Ringe JD, Faber H, Farahmand P, et al. Efficacy of risedronate in men with primary and secondary osteoporosis: results of a 1-year study. Rheumatol Int 2005;7:1–5.

[70] Kaufman JM, Orwoll E, Goemaere S, et al. Teriparatide effects on vertebral fractures and bone mineral density in men with osteoporosis: treatment and discontinuation of therapy. Osteoporos Int 2004;16:510–6.

[71] Orwoll ES, Scheele WH, Paul S, et al. The effect of teriparatide (human parathyroid hormone [1–34]) therapy on bone density in men with osteoporosis. J Bone Miner Res 2003; 18:9–17.

[72] Kurland ES, Cosman F, McMahon DJ, et al. Parathyroid hormone as a therapy for idiopathic osteoporosis in men: effects on bone mineral density and bone markers. J Clin Endocrinol Metab 2000;85:3069–76.

[73] Finkelstein JS, Hayes A, Hunzelman JL, et al. The effects of parathyroid hormone, alendronate, or both in men with osteoporosis. N Engl J Med 2003;349:1216–26.

[74] Lim GC, Moses AM. Resistance to the action of vitamin D in mother and daughter with asymptomatic celiac disease. Presented at the 87th Annual Meeting of the Endocrine Society. San Diego, June 4, 2005.

[75] Kuehn BM. Longer-lasting osteoporosis drugs sought. JAMA 2005;293:2458.

[76] Vermeulen A. Androgen replacement therapy in the aging male-a critical evaluation. J Clin Endocrinol Metab 2001;86:2380–90.

[77] Rosen CJ, Bilezikian JP. Clinical review 123: hot topic anabolic therapy for osteoporosis. J Clin Endocrinol Metab 2001;86:957–64.

[78] Miller PD, Bilezikian JP, Deal C, et al. Clinical use of the teriparatide in the real world: initial insights. Endocr Pract 2004;2:139–48.

[79] Epstein S. The roles of bone mineral density, bone turnover, and other properties in reducing fracture risk during antiresorptive therapy. Mayo Clin Proc 2005;80:379–88.

[80] Felsenberg D, Boonen S. The bone quality framework: determinants of bone strength and their interrelationships, and implications for osteoporosis management. Clin Ther 2005; 27:1–11.

NURSING
CLINICS
OF NORTH AMERICA

ELSEVIER
SAUNDERS

Nurs Clin N Am 42 (2007) 101–111

Pheochromocytoma: Challenges in Diagnosis and Nursing Care

Katharyn F. Daub, EdD, CTN, CNE, RN

Department of Baccalaureate Nursing, University of Hawaii at Hilo,
200 West Kawili Street, Hilo, HI 96720, USA

Pheochromocytomas are catecholamine-secreting tumors arising from chromaffin cells of the sympathoadrenal system, which includes the adrenal medulla and sympathetic ganglionic tissue. The effects of catecholamine excess cause potentially fatal symptomologies and end-organ damage if not diagnosed and treated; however, if diagnosed and removed surgically, most patients can be cured. Pheochromocytomas are rare, affecting from two to eight per million people [1]. There are 800 deaths in the United States annually as a result of complications. Of patients who have pheochromocytomas diagnosed at autopsy, 75% died suddenly from myocardial infarction or cerebral vascular catastrophe [2]. Challenges in diagnosis, tumor location, and treatment are considerable.

Definitions and epidemiology

Catecholamine-secreting tumors may arise in the adrenal medulla (pheochromocytoma) or in extra-adrenal chromaffin cells (paraganglioma) [3]. Chromaffin cells are named because of their affinity for chromium salts as a staining method for microscopy. This was an early method of detecting these cells [2]. This rare tumor affects only 0.2% of patients who have documented hypertension [4]. Most pheochromocytomas occur sporadically and are located in the adrenal medulla (90%). The "rule of tens" has been used to define the various types of pheochromocytomas: 10% pediatric, 10% extra-adrenal, 10% familial, 10% pediatric, 10% bilateral (renal), and 10% multiple [5,6]. Extra-adrenal pheochromocytomas or paragangliomas occur most commonly in the so-called "organ of Zukerkandl" (75%), but also can be found in the thorax, pelvis, mediastinum, and neck [5,7]. With

E-mail address: katharyn@hawaii.edu

paragangliomas, recurrences are increased up to 11-fold [3]. Accounting for the 10% of familial disorders are multiple endocrine neoplasia type IIA (MEN-IIA) and von Hippel–Lindau disease. MEN-IIA is characterized by the familial association of medullary thyroid cancer, pheochromocytoma, and parathyroid hyperplasia. Patients who have von Hippel–Lindau disease develop early-onset bilateral kidney tumors, pheochromocytomas, cerebellar and spinal hemangioblastomas, retinal angiomas, and pancreatic cysts and tumors [8].

Clinical presentation

Patients who have pheochromocytoma present with the signs and symptoms of catecholamine excess, including epinephrine, norepinephrine, and dopamine [4,5]. Paroxysms (spells) are the classic feature of pheochromocytoma. They begin abruptly, last from minutes to hours, subside gradually, with a frequency that varies from many times daily, to one or more per week, or even one every 2 months [9]. Hypertension, sometimes dangerously elevated, is seen often with pheochromocytoma. Sustained hypertension occurs in 50% of patients, paroxysmal hypertension occurs in 30% of patients, and normotension occurs in less than 20% of patients. A classic triad of symptoms—episodic headaches, sweating, and palpitations—has been described [5]. Many other nonspecific signs and symptoms may occur, such as pallor, anxiety, flushing, visual blurring, polyuria, polydipsia, hyperglycemia, weight loss, papilledema, orthostatic hypotension, and decreased gastrointestinal motility. In addition, tachydysrhythmias, myocarditis, stroke, dilated cardiomyopathy, and myocardial infarction may be evident. The diagnosis may be delayed, given the fact that pheochromocytomas are rare, the symptomology is not specific, and the tumor may remain silent for long periods of time, because catecholamines can be converted to inactive metanephrines within the tumor [3]. The clinician needs to use his or her skills in history taking and physical assessment to develop a suspicion, because delay in diagnosis or misdiagnosis can cause considerable morbidity or mortality. Pheochromocytomas should be considered in patients who have labile hypertension or hypertension that is resistant to therapy [10].

Other causes of sympathetic overactivity need to be considered. Autonomic dysfunction, as in Guillain-Barré syndrome, or post–spinal cord injury will increase sympathetic activity. Panic and other stress responses produce symptoms that are due to increased sympathetic activity. The use of sympathomimetic drugs (ie, phenylpropanolamine, cocaine, amphetamines, epinephrine, phenylephrine, turbutaline) increase circulating catecholamines. Also, the combination of monoamine oxidase inhibitors and tyramine-containing foods can produce absorption of tyramine that increases the release of norepinephrine from nerve endings and epinephrine from adrenal glands [4]. Examples of foods that are high in tyramines are fermented cheeses, Chianti wine, champagne, other wines, soy sauce, avocados, bananas, overripe foods, and any smoked fish or meat.

The abnormalities in carbohydrate metabolism that occur are related directly to the increase in production of catecholamines. Epinephrine-induced glycogen breakdown occurs in the liver, which causes an increase in serum glucose [11]. Catecholamines also decrease insulin secretion from the pancreas and increase lipolysis from adipose tissue, which increases serum lipids.

Biochemical diagnosis

The diagnosis of pheochromocytoma is based on measuring excessive amounts of catecholamines and their metabolites in the urine or plasma. There is debate on the best biochemical screening method. The plasma fractionated metanephrines test is highly sensitive and easy to perform; however, there is approximately 15% false positive readings [5,10,11]. The gold standard for pheochromocytoma diagnosis has been the 24-hour urine for total metanephrines, catecholamines, and vanillylmandelic acid (VMA), which is associated with fewer false positive results [1]. Whichever method is used, a diagnosis of pheochromocytoma can be made with elevated biochemical assays. Some medications may cause false positive results for catecholamines and metanephrines (Box 1) [12,13].

If possible, these drugs should be avoided 5 days before the examination. Drug influence can occur by interfering with the assay in vitro or by causing changes in catecholamine levels directly [12]. Foods to avoid for 1 day before the test include caffeine, alcohol, nicotine, bananas, vanilla, and

---

Box 1. Medications that may cause false positive results for catecholamines and metanephrines

Acetaminophen
Benzodiazepines
Buspirone
Catecholamines
Diuretics
Labetalol
Levodopa
Metoclopramide
Methyldopa
Sympathomimetics
Tricyclic antidepressants
Vasodilators

chocolate [13]. It is important for nurses to identify medications in the patient health history that may have implications related to pheochromocytoma diagnosis. Also major physical stress, including surgery, sleep apnea, myocardial infarction, or ketoacidosis, can cause false positive results [11]. Hypoglycemia also is an important consideration, because epinephrine is secreted vigorously in response to mobilize liver glycogen.

Proper urine collection is important to assure accurate results. Patients must be instructed in detail on collection of specimens. Urine should be collected only in the plastic 24-hour urine container, and stored in a cool, dark place. The test should be delayed for women during menstruation [13].

Locating tumor

Once the biochemical diagnosis of pheochromocytoma has been made, the next task is to locate the tumor. Generally, CT scans or MRI scans are used. Most of these tumors are found on the adrenal gland, which is identified easily on these scans; however, if the adrenal glands appear normal, then the search for an extra-adrenal paraganglioma ensues. Sometimes, the astute radiologist can pick up a paraganglioma along the sympathetic chain; however, many times other modalities need to be used. In either case, an ^{123}I-metaiodobenzylguanidine (MIBG) scintigraphy can detect tumors that are not detected by CT or MRI, or multiple tumors when CT or MRI is positive [4]. In addition, MIBG is indicated in patients with large adrenal pheochromocytomas (> 10 cm) or paraganglioma, because of the increased risk for multiple tumors or malignancy [4].

Surgical treatment

In the preoperative setting, there are several mandatory requirements to provide for a safe surgical outcome. An α-blocker, usually phenoxybenzamine, is given for 7 to 10 days preoperatively to normalize blood pressure and to expand the contractive blood volumes [4]. A high-sodium diet is prescribed at this time to aid in the intravascular volume expansion. After α-blockade, β-blockade is initiated 2 to 3 days preoperatively for heart rate control. The β-adrenergic blocker should not be started first because blockade of vasodilatory peripheral β-receptors with unopposed α-stimulation can lead to a further dangerous elevation in blood pressure [4,14]. An important part of the nursing care plan at this time is patient care conferences that include family members, because anxiety related to surgical outcome is of concern.

With most sporadic adrenal pheochromocytomas, laparoscopic lateral transabdominal adrenalectomy is the preferred operation for benign-appearing pheochromocytomas of the adrenal glands [5,15]. Indications for open adrenalectomy are tumor size (> 8–10 cm), periadrenal fibrosis, or evidence of local invasion or recurrent tumor [5]. Paragangliomas require an open exploratory procedure because of the difficult location of the sympathetic ganglia. These are high-risk surgical procedures that require an experienced surgical and anesthesia team. Direct arterial pressure monitoring and central pressure monitoring are required. An acute hypertensive crisis may occur before or during the operation and can be treated with nitroprusside [4]. Although preoperative planning for increased intravascular volume was undertaken, there is still the risk for hypotensive episodes after removal of the tumor; generally, these are responsive to intravenous fluid replacement. In a retrospective Mayo Clinic study, few patients who had pheochromocytoma or paraganglioma experienced significant perioperative morbidity, and none died in this largest study to date [16].

The postoperative period requires close cardiovascular monitoring because catecholamine levels can remain high for several days. Hypertension can be treated with nitroprusside or other antihypertensives, and hypotension is responsive to saline infusion with the guidance of central pressure monitoring. With the decrease in circulating catecholamines and the resultant increase in insulin production, close monitoring of serum glucose by the nurse is warranted [9].

Surgical removal does not always lead to a long-term cure, even in patients who have a benign tumor. Up to one third of patients remain hypertensive, despite normal catecholamines, as a result of renal vascular damage [17]. Recurrence is more likely in patients who have familial pheochromocytomas, right adrenal tumors, or paraganglioma. Urinary catecholamines and metanephrines should be measured 2 weeks after resection of the tumor; elevated levels suggest a second tumor that was not identified on initial localization [18]. In addition, long-term monitoring is indicated in all patients, and most should have an annual biochemical screening. Thus, an important inclusion in discharge teaching is the importance of long-term follow-up screening [4].

Malignancy

Malignant chromaffin cell tumors account for 10% to 20% of all pheochromocytomas [19]. It is impossible to determine whether a pheochromocytoma is malignant from histologic appearance [14]. No preoperative data can reliably differentiate between benign and malignant pheochromocytoma [20]. Malignant status is established upon evidence of local invasion or distant metastasis at nonchromaffin sites [8,21]. Malignant tumors may become apparent as long as 15 years after resection [4]. Most metastases are found in lymph nodes, bone, liver, and lung tissues [14]. The ^{131}I-MIBG scintigraphy is used to identify metastatic sites, and can be used to treat inoperable malignant pheochromocytomas and paragangliomas. Pheochromocytomas and paragangliomas that demonstrate positive uptake on a diagnostic MIBG scan can be treated with ^{131}I-MIBG in the patient with metastasis, with palliation of symptoms, reduction of tumor function, as well as tumor arrest or even regression with substantial improvement in the quality of life [5,19]. Metastatic lesions should be resected if possible. Skeletal metastatic lesions can be treated with radiation therapy. If the tumor is aggressive and the quality of life declines, chemotherapy can be considered. Hypertension and spells can be treated with α- and β-blockade. The 5-year survival rate for patients who have malignant pheochromocytoma is 50%.

New developments

Currently, mutations in at least six distinct genes have been associated with predisposition of these tumors, and additional pheochromocytoma-causing genes are likely to be identified [21,22]. Recent work has suggested that tendency to malignancy can be linked to genetic determinants. Advances in the understanding of tumor formation can pave the way for future therapeutic modalities [21].

^{18}F-DA positron emission tomography (PET) was shown to be superior to ^{131}I-MIBG scintigraphy in the location of disease sites in patients who had metastatic pheochromocytoma [23]. As PET scanning becomes more accessible, undoubtedly it will be used more often for this purpose.

With the increase and improvements in abdominal imaging scans for various purposes, there has been an increase in adrenal incidentalomas, defined as a "mass lesion serendipitously discovered by radiologic examination, in the absence of symptoms or clinical findings suggestive of adrenal disease" [6]. All patients who have incidental adrenal tumors should be screened biochemically for pheochromocytoma [8].

Case study

Homer was a 42-year-old man, who in the past 5 years had developed diastolic hypertension, palpitations, an exorbitant increase in his lipid profile, and mild hyperglycemia. He had been started on diltiazem for blood pressure control with little success, and was switched to metoprolol, also without success. He was counseled to reduce his fat intake, his coffee intake, and his alcohol consumption, all of which he complied with. Despite these efforts, his hypertension became more severe, laboratory studies continued to deteriorate, and the palpitations became more frequent, more severe, and more debilitating. When he went to the emergency room because of severe palpitations associated with diaphoresis and light headedness, he was noted to be in a rapid atrial fibrillation, with a rate of more than 200 beats per minute, a blood pressure of 240/140 mm Hg, and a pounding headache. His oxygenation was adequate, although he reported shortness of breath. This episode had started several hours earlier and seemed unrelenting. The patient was anxious and had a feeling of impending doom.

The emergency room staff administered oxygen, drew blood for a cardiac work-up, obtained a 12-lead EKG, and started an intravenous infusion of diltiazem for rate control and blood pressure reduction. Homer denied drug use, but a urine sample for drug screen was obtained. Gradually, over the course of the next hour, Homer's blood pressure and heart rate were reduced to acceptable levels; within 2 hours, he was in a normal sinus rhythm with a rate of 70 beats per minute and a blood pressure of 140/100 mm Hg. His other symptoms had resolved. His cardiac laboratory work-up was unremarkable; his 12-lead EKG showed diffuse lateral ST depression and T-wave changes that resolved over the course of his emergency room stay.

Homer was admitted to the ICU for monitoring and serial cardiac enzyme studies. Blood was sent for a complete thyroid panel. An echocardiogram revealed left ventricular hypertrophy. Homer's drug screen was negative for any stimulant drugs of abuse. His condition remained stable overnight as the 24-hour urine collection for catecholamines and metanephrines and VMA was initiated. When questioned as to the episodic nature of his symptoms, Homer stated that he had had similar episodes for several years, but not as severe and long lasting as this episode. The spells always subsided spontaneously.

Homer was released from the hospital 2 days later having submitted his 24-hour urine and finding out that all of his thyroid tests and cardiac tests had come back normal. He was to follow-up with his physician in 2 days; in the meantime, Homer was placed on an increased dose of diltiazem, one aspirin a day, and a statin for his dyslipidemia.

On his follow-up visit, Homer was confronted with a frightening diagnosis. His doctor informed him that he had a biochemically diagnosed pheochromocytoma, primarily secreting large amounts of norepinephrine (three times normal) as well as epinephrine. The doctor explained that this was good news, because if this condition continued it was likely to cause bigger problems in the future. He explained that treatment for a pheochromocytoma is surgical excision and that his chances of recovery were good. Homer's first question was, "Is that tumor cancer?". The doctor explained that there was no way to tell now, but there was a 10% chance that it could be malignant. Homer did not know whether to be relieved or panic stricken.

The next step was to find Homer's tumor. He went for an abdominal CT scan. The doctors said that this test would show up to 90% of pheochromocytoma tumors. Unfortunately for Homer, the CT was read as normal, placing him in the 10% of patients who have an extra-adrenal pheochromocytoma or paraganglioma. This makes the work-up more difficult and the surgery more extensive. Next on the list was an MRI scan of the chest, abdomen, and pelvis. Again, this was a negative finding for pheochromocytoma. Homer was beginning to get discouraged, having read on the Internet the various possibilities of paragangliomas and metastatic lesions. His doctor reassured him that the next test would focus directly on his tumor, the ^{131}I-MIBG scintigraphy. After two sessions in the nuclear medicine department, the radiologist gave Homer the good news that his tumor had been found. Examination demonstrated a bilobed focus of abnormal activity in the retroperitoneum, just anterior to the spine at the level of the distal aorta, measuring 6 cm × 2.5 cm. This location, the so-called "organ of Zuckerkandl," was the most common location of a very uncommon tumor (Fig. 1). The radiologist was able to confirm his diagnosis on the CT scan, where he found it retrospectively.

Homer was referred to a large tertiary medical center and a surgical team that was experienced in resection of extra-adrenal pheochromocytomas. In preparation for surgery, Homer was placed on phenoxybenzamine and encouraged to eat as much salt as he wanted. This was done to increase intravascular volume before surgery and to control blood pressure. He was orthostatic at first, and had to stand up slowly. Also, he had a stuffy nose, which is the other classic side effect of phenoxybenzamine. He adhered religiously to the doctor's instruction of increasing his salt intake. Two days preoperatively, he was started on propanolol for heart rate control. A preoperative echocardiogram, chest radiograph, EKG, repeat catecholamine studies on serum and urine, multitudes of laboratory studies, and a physical evaluation by the attending Endocrinologist were performed. In addition,

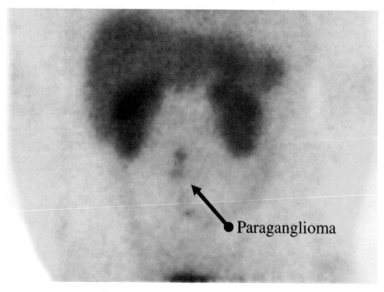

Fig. 1. ^{131}I-MIBG scintigraphy showing paraganglioma.

Homer met a nurse practitioner who would follow him from his preoperative phase to discharge.

The surgery was performed with an arterial line in place, central lines, lots of fluids hanging, and a nipride drip ready to go. Intubation and induction of anesthesia went without problems, which was a relief because this can stimulate a catecholamine crisis. A primary long midline incision was made, and the peritoneal cavity was entered sharply. Exploration revealed the liver, gall bladder, pancreas, stomach, small bowel, and colon to be essentially normal. The bowel was elevated, which afforded excellent visualization of the aorta and vena cava, with the overlying dumb-bell–shaped, hard, well-circumscribed paraganglioma (Fig. 2). Eventually, it was excised intact and sent to pathology. Palpation along the remainder of the aorta and inferior vena cava did not reveal any additional sites of tumor. When removing the tumor, there was modest elevation in Homer's blood pressure, and when it was removed completely, fluid was given to restore modest hypotension.

Postoperatively, Homer's course was uneventful, with the exception of hypoglycemia the first night, which was treated with intravenous dextrose. This was due to his decreasing circulating catecholamines and the resultant increasing insulin secretion. Homer's 24-hour urine for catecholamines and metanephrines done 2 days postoperatively was negative; he left the hospital on the third postoperative day.

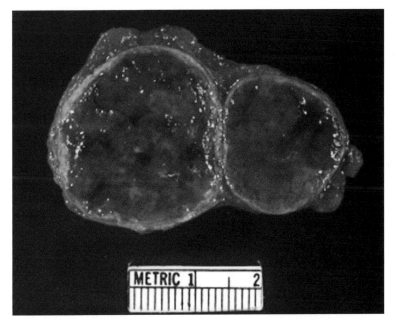

Fig. 2. Paraganglioma: inferior vena cava region.

Today, Homer is normotensive, has a normal lipid profile, no longer has hyperglycemia, and is only taking an aspirin daily. Because he had a paraganglioma, annual biochemical screenings for catecholamines or metanephrines will be done indefinitely.

Summary

Since the first pheochromocytoma was resected by Dr. Charles Mayo in 1926, without the aid of diagnostic testing and imaging, many important technologic advances have occurred that make finding and treating these rare tumors more straightforward. From biochemical testing for catecholamines and metanephrines to the sophisticated imaging and nuclear medicine diagnostics, medical science has assembled much to improve patient outcome.

Despite all of the technologic advances, saving a patient who has a pheochromocytoma depends mainly on a health care professional, with an index of suspicion, screening for this tumor before it causes significant morbidity or even death.

References

[1] Kudva H, Sawka A, Young W. The laboratory diagnosis of adrenal pheochromocytoma: The Mayo Clinic Experience. J Clin Endocrinol Metab 2003;88(10):4532–9.
[2] Clark O, Duh Q-Y, editors. The textbook of endocrine surgery. 1st edition. Philadelphia: WB Saunders; 1977.
[3] Amar L, Servais A, Gimenez-Roqueplo AP, et al. Year of diagnosis, features at presentation, and risk of recurrence in patients with pheochromocytoma or secreting paraganglioma. J Clin Endocrinol Metab 2005;90(4):2110–6.
[4] Young W, Kaplan N. Diagnosis and treatment of pheochromocytoma in adults. Available at: http://uptodateonline.com/utd/content/topic.do?topicKey=adrenal/19691&view=text. Accessed April 21, 2006.
[5] Yeo H, Roman S. Pheochromocytoma and functional paraganglioma. Curr Opin Oncol 2005;17(1):13–8.
[6] Yogish C, Young W, Thompson G, et al. Adrenal incidentaloma: an important component of the clinical presentation spectrum of benign sporadic adrenal pheochromocytoma. Endocrinologist 1999;9(9):77–80.
[7] Whalen RF, Althausen AF, Daniels GH. Extra-adrenal pheochromocytoma. Br J Surg 1987;74:7.
[8] Torrey S. Recognition and management of adrenal emergencies. Emerg Med Clin North Am 2005;23(3):687–702 , vii.
[9] Goldman L, Bennett C, editors. The adrenal medulla, catecholamines, and pheochromocytoma, 21st edition (Cecil Textbook of Medicine). Philadelphia: WB Saunders; 2000.
[10] Norman A, Litwack G, editors. Hormones of the adrenal medulla. 2nd edition (Hormones). San Diego (CA): Academic Press; 1997.
[11] Eisenhofer G, Goldstein D, McClellan M, et al. Endocrine care of special interest to the practice of endocrinology. J Clin Endocrinol Metab 2003;88(16):2110–6.
[12] Westphal S. Diagnosis of a pheochromocytoma. Am J Med Sci 2005;329(1):18–21.

[13] Capital Health. Available at: http://www.capitalhealth.ca/AboutUs/OurOrganization/AreasolService/LaboratoryMedicine. Accessed June 24, 2006.

[14] Young W. Pheochromocytoma: 1926–1993. Trends Endocrinol Metab 1993;4(4):122–7.

[15] Tobias-Machado M, Rincon Rios F, Tulio Lasmar M, et al. Laparoscopic retroperitoneal adrenalectomy as a minimally invasive option for the treatment of adrenal tumors. Arch Esp Urol 2006;59(1):49–54.

[16] Kinney M, Warner M, vanHeerden J, et al. Perianesthetic risks and outcomes of pheochromocytoma and paraganglioma resection. Anesth Analg 2000;91(5):1118–23.

[17] Burton M. Emergency! Pheochromocytoma. Am J Nurs 1997;97(11):57.

[18] Goldstein RE, O'Neill JA, Holcomb GW. Clinical experience over 48 years with pheochromocytoma. Ann Surg 1999;229:755–66.

[19] Kaltsas G, Mukherjee J, Foley R, et al. Treatment of metastatic pheochromocytoma and paraganglioma with 131I-Meta-Iodobenzylguanidine (MIBG). Endocrinologist 2003;13(4):321–33.

[20] Lombardi CP, Raffaelli M, De Crea C, et al. Pheochromocytoma: role of preoperative diagnosis in the assessment of malignancy risk and in the choice of surgical approach. Suppl Tumori 2005;4(3):S211.

[21] Dahia P. Evolving concepts in pheochromocytoma and paraganglioma. Curr Opin Oncol 2006;18(1):1–8.

[22] Benn D, Gimenez-Roqueplo A, Reilly J, et al. Clinical presentation and penetrance of pheochromocytoma/paraganglioma syndromes. J Clin Endocrinol Metab 2006;91(3):827–36.

[23] Ilias I, Yu J, Carrasquillo J, et al. Superiority of 6-[18F]-fluorodopamine positron emission tomography versus [131I]-metaiodobenzylguanidine scintigraphy in the localization of metastatic pheochromocytoma. J Clin Endocrinol Metab 2003;88(9):4083–7.

NURSING
CLINICS
OF NORTH AMERICA

Nurs Clin N Am 42 (2007) 113–125

Diabetes and Thyroid Disease: Nursing Care to Improve Outcomes for Patients Living in Poverty

Julie Miller, RN, MSN

MedCentral College of Nursing, 335 Glessner Avenue, Mansfield, OH 44903, USA

A primary goal of nurses providing care for persons who have diabetes mellitus or thyroid disease is improving the health outcomes for those persons. Improving health outcomes for these individuals can seem a daunting task when considering all elements of the care process, let alone all of the differences in the lives of those individuals. The process for care of the individual who has diabetes or thyroid disease is similar: assessment/diagnosis, care planning, treatment/interventions, and management/evaluation. This process of care is improved for individuals when there is an understanding of the disease and an understanding demonstrated by the nurse of "where those individuals come from" (ie, socioeconomic status [SES], educational level, race, ethnicity). For persons who have diabetes or thyroid disease and live in poverty, improving the care process, and ultimately health outcomes, must include the nurse's understanding of poverty. The purpose of this article is to provide nurses with a basic understanding of the resource issues, "hidden rules," and characteristics that are associated with persons who live in poverty. Most importantly, some basic strategies to improve the health outcomes of patients who have diabetes or thyroid disease and live in poverty are provided.

The first step toward improving health outcomes for persons who have diabetes or thyroid disease is to have a basic understanding of the scope of these diseases and their relationship to poverty in the United States. The number of Americans who have diabetes has more than doubled over the last 20 years, from 5.8 million to 14.7 million. Unfortunately, the United States also has the largest number of diabetics of all the developed countries in the world [1]. It is estimated that by the year 2025, approximately 22 million Americans will have diabetes [2]. Although any portion of the

E-mail address: jmiller@medcentral.edu

population can be impacted by diabetes, the disease can be tremendously taxing to certain groups, including those living in poverty or in a lower SES [3]. SES, as measured by individual or household income, education, employment, occupation, or living in an underprivileged area, has been associated with poor glycemic control and related glycemic control health issues [4].

Thyroid disease, in comparison, impacts the lives of approximately 20 million Americans. This disease, although similar to diabetes in that it can affect any portion of the population, is tremendously taxing to women and even more so to women of lower SES [5].

There is little research available that focuses specifically on thyroid disease and SES; however, a myriad of information is available on the relationship of poverty to diabetes and other chronic diseases. Poverty has been associated with increased risks for cardiovascular disease, respiratory disease, ulcers, rheumatoid disorders, psychiatric diseases, and several types of cancers [6]. Individuals living in poverty are taxed more often by those chronic and disabling diseases because of issues related to such things as the availability and accessibility of quality health care, delay in seeking treatment, inability to pay for health care services, and lack of basic health care knowledge, among others. Poverty also affects lifestyle factors that play a role in chronic illness. Individuals may live in substandard housing that is cold, damp, and filthy. Diet and nutrition may be inappropriate and can contribute to poor diabetic control, obesity, and heart disease. In addition, simply getting to the doctor may be difficult without a flexible work or childcare schedule, let alone the transportation needed to get there. A tremendous challenge for nurses in the United States is gaining an understanding of disparities in health. There also is a need to better understand the links between poverty and these disparities; however, many key decision makers (ie, politicians) still seem to believe that chronic illnesses afflict only the affluent and the elderly and that these illnesses arise only from freely accepted and acquired risks. They also believe that the control of chronic diseases should not be considered a high priority (unlike infectious disease, which garners a wealth of respect and public attention). These beliefs are based on false assumptions about the chronic disease burden.

Although the disease burden is more variable in developing countries, the poorest populations, particularly in rapidly growing United States cities, already exhibit the highest risks for tobacco use, alcohol use, and physical inactivity, with evidence emerging for obesity. This will produce a higher burden of chronic diseases over the long-term. Poverty also leads to greater comorbidity because of a decreased access to quality medical care [7]. In addition, it often is difficult for many health care providers to accept that in the United States, many individuals live in conditions similar to those of the direst poverty of developing countries [8]. However, as stated by Neil Calman [9] in his report: *Making Health Equality a Reality: The Bronx Takes Action* "although the determinants of health disparities are complex and varied, we do not need to unravel every last piece of this puzzle to begin to take action." Therefore, although a complete understanding of the relationship between poverty and chronic health issues, such as diabetes and thyroid disease, has not been fully elucidated, nurses must begin to "take action" by developing an understanding of poverty and how it affects the health and health care of those who live in and with it.

Understanding resources

The American Heritage Dictionary [10] defines poverty as "the state of being poor; lack of the means of providing material needs or comforts." An individual's ability or inability to provide for material needs or comforts certainly impact his or her quality of life. Dr. Ruby Payne, author of *A Framework for Understanding Poverty*, defines quality of life by the degree to which an individual possesses 10 essential resources (Table 1).

As defined above, poverty seems to be relative. For the purposes of this article, however, "poverty" is defined as the extent to which an individual lives without resources [11]. The focus is on individuals living with a lack of financial resources or in economic poverty. Although all of the resources will be considered, economic poverty or class is the focus because of the impact that financial resources have on many of the other essential resources and on quality of life. Economic poverty occurs in all races and in all

Table 1
Resources

Resource	Defining characteristics
Financial	Having the money to purchase goods and services, and an understanding of how money works
Emotional	Possessing the ability not to be self-destructive in negative situations, being able to control and choose emotions
Physical	Enjoying physical health and mobility
Mental	Being able to read, write, and compute
Spiritual	Believing in a divine purpose or guidance
Relationships/role models	Possessing access to people who are appropriate, nurturing, and who are not self-destructive
Support systems	Having social networks of support that often are people outside of a person's inner circle—this can be groups or businesses
Motivation, persistence	Experiencing the energy or drive to plan and complete such things as projects, jobs, and life changes
Integrity, trust	Trust is related to predictability and safety. Can I safely say that this person/agency is trustworthy and that they act consistently? Is it safe for me to be with them?
Knowledge of hidden rules	Knowledge of the hidden rules of poverty, middle class, and wealth

From Payne RK, DeVol P, Dreussi-Smith T. Bridges out of poverty: strategies for professionals and communities. Highlands (TX): aha!process, Inc.; 2001; with permission.

countries; economic class is a continuous line, not a clear-cut distinction. In-dividuals are found all along the continuum of income, and sometimes they move up or down on that continuum. There also is a difference between "generational poverty" and "situational poverty." Generational poverty is defined by Payne and colleagues [11] as being in economic poverty for two generations or longer. Situational poverty has a shorter time frame and is caused by such things as divorce, sickness, death, or a lack of neces-sary resources. In summary, generational, economic poverty is the "culture" or class identified in this article.

To gain a better understanding of the relationship between resources and poverty consider the following case study.

Juanita is a perimenopausal, Latino mother of six children. The youngest child weighed more than 9 pounds at birth and is now 4 years old. The other children are of elementary school age. Juanita's family recently emigrated from Mexico. They are living in a mobile home, located in a poor area, iso-lated from any urban communities. Juanita walked 5 miles to a public clinic with her 4-year-old because she was not feeling well. She presented to the clinic at the age of 47, with limited English language skills, and reported symptoms of polyuria for 2 weeks and excessive thirst for approximately 1 month. It also was seen that she had a massive staphylococcus impetigo. She reported to the nurse practitioner (NP) that she was quenching her thirst with canned Coca Cola, which her husband had stolen from his employer, because she did not have a sanitary water supply; that her only income was her husband's minimum wage salary at the local brick yard; and that she was uninsured. A random blood glucose was drawn and found to be 453 mg/dL (normal, 70–125 mg/dL) and her hemoglobin A1c was 18 (nor-mal, $\leq$7%). The NP was unable to admit Juanita to the hospital; they would not take her because she could not pay for her care. The NP made the decision to give Juanita some metformin (Glucophage) samples, take her off the cola, and to give her a 1- or 2-day supply of bottled water, an injection of penicillin, and some Penicillin VK tablets. The NP asked Juanita to return the following morning for a fasting blood sugar and a 2-hour post-prandial blood sugar (with a 100-g load). Surprising to the NP, Juanita re-turned the next morning; tests revealed a fasting blood sugar of 212 mg/dL (normal, 70–99 mg/dL) and a 2-hour postprandial blood sugar of 206 mg/dL (normal, 70–145 mg/dL). Oral hypoglycemics, a 2100-calorie diabetic diet, and a dilated eye examination were prescribed.

To begin formulating a plan of care, the nurse should begin by asking "What resources does Juanita seem to have?". Consider which resources you believe are very low, which resources are visible but not adequate, and if the resources available to the patient are adequate to function in the United States health care system. There may not be enough information in the case study for one to make a full determination; however, it is obvious that Juanita has limited (some but not enough) financial resources (ie, her husband works a minimum wage job, she has no health insurance, and there is a family of eight to feed). Of equal importance is the lack of resources related to her lack of understanding and speaking of the English language, limited support system resources due to her recent immigration to the United States, and limited integrity and trust resources because she is visiting a new clinic and new health care provider in a new country. She may have limited physical resources if the elevated blood glucose levels have led to complications. Juanita also must learn how to adapt to a health care system that has a set of "hidden rules" that she does not yet understand. There are no right or wrong answers to this case study. This case study illustrates a situation in health care that too often arises for people with limited resources: the inability to get the quality of health care that is needed as evidenced by the hospital not admitting the patient, limitations in access to health care because of limited transportation or childcare issues, and the inability to pay for needed health resources (eg, medicines, clean water).

Some of the resources presented are internal, coming from inside the individual. Some resources are external, coming from the community, friends, or family. Some of the resources are internal and external. No one individual can build resources on one's own, and the use and improvement of the resources is determined individually [12].

When considering resources, nurses and other health care professionals first must determine that the problems that an individual is facing are not the result of a systems issue. This means that it must be determined that Juanita's delay in obtaining timely health care was not a result of clinic hours or how clinic appointments are scheduled. Once it is determined that system issues are not the cause, the individual's resources should be assessed. Nurses should avoid accusing individuals, and instead, attempt to assess and understand the individual's available resources, strengths, and weaknesses. What may seem like workable solutions to the nurse who works in a typical American, middle-class setting may be extremely difficult for an individual living in poverty given the resources that one possesses.

Understanding hidden rules

Hidden rules are the unspoken cues and habits of a group [11]. Between and among groups and economic classes there is a specific system for cueing. This generally is recognized for racial and ethnic groups in the United States, but typically not for socioeconomic class. Health care facilities in the United States operate from "middle-class" norms and use the hidden rules of the middle class. Understanding the hidden rules of a client's SES is extremely important. Hidden rules exist in poverty, in middle-class, and in wealth, as well as in racial and ethnic groups. There are hidden rules about dress, manners, and food in each of the classes. If an individual has been raised in and lives in the middle class, he/she will understand the hidden rules of the middle class, and typically will assume that everyone understands those rules. Similarly, if an individual has been raised in and lives in poverty, he/she will understand the hidden rules of the poverty class, and typically will assume that everyone understands those rules. If a nurse who understands only the hidden rules of the middle class works with an individual who understands only the hidden rules of the poverty class, the chances that the individual will achieve optimal health care outcomes are limited. It is important for nurses who work with individuals from poverty to understand the hidden rules of poverty, and to be willing to teach the hidden rules of the health care agency/system for which they work. Understanding and teaching will provide the opportunity for success in meeting health care outcomes. The relationship must be reciprocal.

A major issue facing the nurse caring for diabetic clients living in poverty is that of appropriate diet. It is known that an appropriate diet is a cornerstone to achieving optimal glycemic level control. Consider, however, the situation faced by those living without a predictable income. There are concerns about not having enough food. Some weeks there is plenty of food, whereas during other weeks the food has to be stretched. Those in poverty also have to concern themselves with the quality of the food that they can afford. A study in the *American Journal of Preventive Medicine* [13] reported that 23% of the nation's lower income classes are obese, compared with 16% of the middle and upper classes; that larger supermarket chains (the best bet for affordable, fresh, and healthy foods) have abandoned less affluent city neighborhoods, focusing instead on the suburbs; that a 1997 US Department of Agriculture study found food prices, including those for produce, are, on average, 10% higher in inner city food markets than they are in the suburbs; and that there are three times as many supermarkets in wealthy neighborhoods as in poor ones.

All hidden rules influence behavior; one of the strongest influences is that of economic class. Throughout this article, only three economic classes are discussed. Because hidden rules of economic class are so powerful in determining behavior, it is pertinent that they be understood when a nurse or other health care provider decides to develop a sustainable relationship with a poor client [12]. A key point here is that nurses must understand that hidden rules govern much of their immediate assessment of an individual and his/her skills and capabilities. These factors often are the reasons why individuals are unsuccessful in achieving optimal health outcomes or even accessing health care in the first place.

Understanding characteristics of poverty

Characteristics of poverty are numerous and often change in response to the life activity or life crisis that is occurring. For clarification and understanding, the characteristics of poverty [11] are provided in Box 1.

Box 1. Characteristics of poverty

Background "noise": Almost always the TV is on, no matter what the circumstance. Conversation is participatory, often with more than one person talking at a time.

Importance of personality: Individual personality is what one brings to the setting—because money is not brought. The ability to entertain, tell stories, and have a sense of humor is highly valued.

Significance of entertainment: When one can merely survive, then the respite from the survival is important. In fact, entertainment brings respite.

Importance of relationships: One only has people upon whom to rely, and those relationships are important to survival. One often has favorites.

Matriarchal structure: The mother has the most powerful position in the society if she functions as a caretaker.

Oral-language tradition: Casual register is used for everything.

Survival orientation: Discussion of academic topics is generally not prized. There is little room for the abstract. Discussions center around people and relationships. A job is about making enough money to survive. A job is not about a career (e.g., "I was looking for a job when I found this one").

Identity tied to lover/fighter role for men: The key issue for males is to be a "man." The rules are rigid and a man is expected to work hard physically—and be a lover and a fighter.

Identity tied to rescuer/martyr role for women: A "good" woman is expected to take care of and rescue her man and her children as needed.

Importance of non-verbal/kinesthetic communication: Touch is used to communicate, as are space and non-verbal emotional information.

Ownership of people: People are possessions. There is a great deal of fear and comment about leaving the culture and "getting above your raisings."

Negative orientation: Failure at anything is the source of stories and numerous belittling comments.

Discipline: Punishment is about penance and forgiveness, not change.

Belief in fate: Destiny and fate are the major tenets of the belief system. Choice is seldom considered.

Polarized thinking: Options are hardly ever examined. Everything is polarized; it is one way or the other. These kinds of statements are common: "I quit" and "I can't do it."

(Continued on next page)

Mating dance: The mating dance is about using the body in a sexual way and verbally and subverbally complimenting body parts. If you have few financial resources, the way you sexually attract someone is with your body.

Time: Time occurs only in the present. The future does not exist except as a word. Time is flexible and not measured. Time is often assigned on the basis of the emotional significance and not the actual measured time.

Sense of humor: A sense of humor is highly valued, as entertainment is one of the key aspects of poverty. Humor is almost always about people—either situations that people encounter or things people do to other people.

Lack of order/organization: Many of the homes/apartments of people in poverty are unkempt and cluttered. Devices for organization (files, planners, etc.) don't exist.

Lives in the moment—does not consider future ramifications: Being proactive, setting goals, and planning ahead are not a part of generational poverty. Most of what occurs is reactive and in the moment. Future implications of present actions are seldom considered.

So what does an understanding of these characteristics do for nurses who care for individuals who live in poverty, and how does it impact the individual's success? It is important to have this knowledge of characteristics to direct your care as well as to be aware of the presence and role you could play in the life of an individual from the poverty culture. Understanding the characteristics can promote patience and improve the manner in which a nurse addresses the care planning of an individual who lives in poverty. Not only can a nurse participate in the work of an individual toward optimal health outcomes, a nurse may assist an individual who chooses to leave poverty. The four primary reasons why people leave poverty include a specific talent or skill that provides an opportunity for them, a person who shows them a different way or that they could live differently, a situation so painful that anything would be better, or a goal or vision of something they want to be or have. Many individuals stay in poverty because they do not realize there is any other option—and if they do know, they usually do not have anyone to teach them about resources or hidden rules. Once the nurse has an understanding of the hidden rules, characteristics, and reasons for leaving or staying in poverty, he/she will become a better client advocate, health educator, care provider, and mentor (if desired).

Strategies to improve health outcomes

Almost half of all people with chronic illnesses have multiple conditions. As a result, many managed care and integrated delivery systems have taken a great interest in correcting the many deficiencies in the current management of diseases such as diabetes, heart disease, depression, asthma, and others. Those deficiencies include rushed practitioners not following established practice guidelines, lack of care coordination, lack of active follow-up to ensure the best outcomes, and patients inadequately trained to manage their illnesses. Overcoming these deficiencies will require nothing less than a transformation of health care, from a system that is essentially reactive—responding mainly when a person is sick—to one that is proactive and focused on keeping a person as healthy as possible [14]. As we consider strategies for working with persons who have diabetes or thyroid disease living in poverty, we must consider individual (nurse) strategies and health systems (work place) strategies. Without an assessment and needed changes being made, the opportunity to improve health outcomes for those individuals will be adequate at best. We begin by looking at individual strategies with an understanding that this is not an all-inclusive list but recommendations that have proven successful in health care and social service environments.

Individual strategies

- Build a knowledge base and understanding of the poverty class.
- Recognize that the building of a relationship with the individual is the most important first step in being successful in your work together. Be aware that you may not be the person that develops the best relationship with the client. It may be the receptionist or medical assistant who develops the best relationship with the client. It would be appropriate then to use the receptionist or assistant (within their scope of practice and abilities) to deliver health education or information that the client needs. The idea is that with the knowledge of how important relationships are to people living in poverty, using the staff member with the best relationship most often assists in meeting the client outcomes that are desired.
- Teach the middle class rules of the agency or facility where you care for the client. Actually talk to them if needed about behavior in the waiting room, the appropriate use of cell phones, language, and touch, make them aware of what happens with missed appointments, and guide and educate them about the forms that you have them fill out. The idea here is that this is a teaching–learning moment for the nurse and the client. It actually can help to build a relationship when you are honest, use the "adult" voice, and just help them navigate a new system. It demonstrates your commitment to their success. You also may want them to teach you about the hidden rules in their world, if they do not share them with you first. Clients need to be taught the hidden rules

of middle class, not in denigration of their own but as another set of rules that can be used if they choose.

- Gather resource information during initial visits. This will help the nurse quickly identify the barriers or potential delays in the care-planning process. The nurse may then work with the client to find or enhance the resources that are in place. Gathering resource information can be done quickly and in a basic manner when added to intake or assessment forms. The resources can be listed on the form and information on each of them added by the nurse or other appropriate staff person.
- Assess and consider reorganizing the schedule and the work day. Support systems and relationships can be built between nurses and clients just by making minor adjustments to the agency day, often without additional costs. By adding 5 minutes to each appointment time, there is now more time for relationship building, hidden rule teaching–learning, and improved health outcomes.
- For persons living in poverty, poor health outcomes often are exacerbated by the lack or limited availability of health care services. Knowledge of the primary assistance programs, their benefits, and their scope of coverage is important to the nurse caring for these clients [14]. Nurses also should be familiar with the services unique to their community.
- Every opportunity to screen for potential problems and provide health education on appropriate health issues must be taken. Clients who have diabetes or thyroid disease living in poverty should, as part of their appointment/examination, be screened for all necessary and potential health issues, as well as be provided health education on immunizations, adequate nutrition, prenatal care (when appropriate), dental and eye examinations, safe water, and food practices. Each encounter should be considered an opportunity to check for additional health concerns or problems. If early screening and treatment improve a person's health, the cost of care is reduced (for delayed care) and the clients' financial resources are then improved [15].

Control of diabetes, as well as thyroid disease, is a highly demanding endeavor when working with clients from poverty. It requires substantial vigilance, lifestyle change, medication adherence, and motivation. Those who suffer the most from the diseases often are the least prepared to deal with it. This means that early detection and increased awareness of diabetes and thyroid disease, although important, are not sufficient [16]. All people who are at risk for diabetes or thyroid disease, especially those who live in poverty, must be helped to develop the skills to navigate the middle-class health care system and the skills necessary to prevent or manage the disease. This only can be done with an understanding of client resources, strengths and weaknesses, and the hidden rules by which the client lives.

It also is important for nurses to assess their own skills in working with individuals from poverty. Review the following internal processes in nursing care and assess your skills and strategies. Assess the skills you have or what strategies you use, what skills and strategies you have that could use some enhancement, and what skills or strategies you do not have in place. A quick assessment is an opportunity to improve nursing care (Box 2).

The list of skills or strategies that the nurse may use when working with clients from poverty is not all-inclusive (see Box 2). There are many more

---

Box 2. Internal processes and skills/strategies that can be used to improve nursing care

Creating relationships
  Seek first to understand
  Keep promises
  Use courtesies
  Clarify expectations
  Be willing to apologize
  Be open to feedback
  Show appreciation for humor and entertainment demonstrated
  Respect demands and priorities of relationships
  Use adult voice
  Respect of unique skills/talents of the individual

Assessment
  Be able to use humor
  Add 5 to 10 minutes
  Comment; do not ask direct questions
  Pick the information that you need out of the story that is told
  Be aware of what is omitted from the story

Care Planning
  Use mediation
  Plan backwards
  Require a plan for each step
  Plan at the beginning of each appointment, not the end
  Teach hidden rules

Sanctions
  Provide choices/consequences
  Use metaphor stories

Agency process
  Assist in changing internal processes to serve poverty culture
  Collaborate with other professionals/agencies to help remove barriers
  Schedule for relationship building

strategies that could be discussed, but not in this limited format. Unfortunately, the internal skills or strategies that the nurse may choose to perform or enhance to improve the health outcomes for his/her clients who are diabetic or have thyroid disease can be limited when the health care agency or system is unaware or nonsupportive. Fortunately, health care agencies and systems can use the same tools provided above to improve health outcomes for their clients. There must be support from the administration. Administrators, supervisors, and middle managers must understand and learn about the poverty culture, and, in turn, be willing to learn about new processes and be open and willing to change. Systems change often is difficult and time consuming; however, with a commitment and a focused desire to improve outcomes for clients it can be done. Clinicians (nurses) too, can contribute to a fuller understanding of how best to enhance the quality and effectiveness of care [17]. Once health care systems acknowledge that individuals of lower SES with multiple risk factors are common in the population (and would be even more common if we could account for all of the known risk factors in existence), and recognize the synergistic influences of these co-occurring risk factors on health and health care experiences, there is a clear call for assisting the people in poverty in more comprehensive ways [18].

The information presented in this article has been an attempt to introduce information about the poverty culture to health care professionals (nurses in particular), in the hopes that outcomes for clients living in poverty who are diabetic or have thyroid disease might be improved. Insights into assessing, understanding, and working with clients from poverty have been presented. If this information has done nothing more than challenge the reader to think differently or consider using the information, than the information has done what it was meant to do.

References

[1] National Diabetes Surveillance System. Prevalence of diabetes. Available at: http://www.cdc.gov/diabetes/statistics. Accessed August 31, 2006.
[2] King H, Aubert R, Herman W. Global burden of diabetes: 1995–2025. Diabetes Care 1998; 21:1414–31.
[3] Harris M, Couric C, Reiber G, et al. Diabetes in America. 2nd edition. Washington, DC: National Institutes of Health; 1995.
[4] Brown A, Ettner SL, Piette J, et al. Socioeconomic position and health among persons with diabetes mellitus: a conceptual framework and review of the literature. Epidemiol Rev 2004; 26:63–77.
[5] Cleveland Clinic Health Information Center. Thyroid disease. Available at: http://www.clevelandclinic.org/health/health-info/docs. Accessed August 25, 2006.
[6] Sapolsky RM. Why zebras don't get ulcers: an updated guide to stress, stress-related diseases, and coping. New York: W.H. Freeman & Company; 1998.
[7] Yach D, Hawkes C, Gould CL, et al. The global burden of chronic diseases: overcoming impediments to prevention and control. JAMA 2004;291(21):2616–22.
[8] Sebastian JG, Bushy A. Special populations in the community: advances in reducing health disparities. Gaithersburg, MD: Aspen Publishers, Inc.; 1999.

[9] Calman N. Making health equality a reality: The Bronx takes action. Health Aff 2005;24(2): 491–8.
[10] American Heritage Dictionary. Boston: Houghton Mifflin Company; 2003.
[11] Payne RK, DeVol P, Dreussi-Smith T. Bridges out of poverty: strategies for professionals and communities. Highlands (TX): aha!process, Inc.; 2001.
[12] DeVol P. Using the hidden rules of class to create sustainable communities. Available at: http://www.ahaprocess.com/files/DeVol/UsingtheHiddenRules. Accessed August 21, 2006.
[13] Goodman L. A rotten deal. Self 2003;(December):34–7.
[14] Wagner E. Presentation on the "Chronic Care Model" given at the 2004 Epidemiology, Biostatistics and Clinical Research Methods Summer Session. Available at: www.improvingchroniccare.org/change/index. Accessed on August 31, 2006.
[15] Maurer FA, Smith CM. Community/public health nursing practice: health for families and communities. 3rd edition. St. Louis (MO): Elsevier Health Sciences; 2004.
[16] Black SA. Diabetes, diversity, and disparity: what do we do with evidence? Am J Public Health 2002;92(4):543–7.
[17] Aday L. At risk in America: the health and health care needs of vulnerable populations in the United States. 2nd edition. San Francisco (CA): Jossey-Bass; 2001.
[18] Shi L, Stevens GD. Vulnerable populations in the United States. San Francisco (CA): Jossey-Bass; 2005.

ELSEVIER
SAUNDERS

Nurs Clin N Am 42 (2007) 127–134

NURSING
CLINICS
OF NORTH AMERICA

Rapid and Reversible Alterations in Thyroid Function Tests in Dehydrated Patients

Juan Ybarra, MD, PhD, FACE[a,*],
Sandra Fernandez, RNP, RD[b]

[a]*Instituto de Cardiología Avanzada y Medicina, Centro Médico Teknon,
C/Vilana 12, Barcelona 08022, Spain*
[b]*Resistencia a la Insulina SL, Barcelona, Spain*

A significant number of elderly patients are hospitalized with dehydration that is due to poor oral intake or gastrointestinal or genitourinary losses. This common clinical condition can result in plasma volume contraction (hypovolemia), and often leads, among other things, to increased concentration of circulating plasma proteins. There is experimental [1] and human [2–5] evidence that hypovolemia and hemoconcentration lead to increased plasma levels of the most commonly recognized markers of extracellular fluid volume status (ECFVS) (bound urea nitrogen (BUN), creatinine, uric acid, albumin, hematocrit).

Almost all thyroid hormones in blood are bound to transport proteins, such as thyroxine (T_4)-binding globulin (TBG) ($\sim 80\%$ of T_4 and $\sim 90\%$ of triiodothyronine [T_3]), albumin ($\sim 5\%$ of T4 and T_3), and (T_4-binding) prealbumin (transthyretin) ($\sim 15\%$ of T_4 and $\sim 5\%$ of T_3) [6,7]. Hence, changes in the concentrations of thyroid hormone–binding proteins (ie, secondary to dehydration leading to hypovolemia) profoundly affect the total hormone concentrations in serum [8,9]. This variability in the TBG, albumin, and transthyretin serum concentrations may explain the frequent changes in the total concentrations of thyroid hormones in the absence of thyroid disease. Because more than 99% of circulating thyroid hormones are protein bound, but can be liberated with great rapidity for entry into cells, it is reasonable to postulate that mild to moderate dehydration may lead to hypovolemia and hemoconcentration, and that the latter may lead

---

* Corresponding author.
E-mail address: juanybarra@hotmail.com (J. Ybarra).

nursing.theclinics.com

to alterations in thyroid hormone–binding proteins, and, thus, to alterations in total serum hormone levels.

The current clinical study was designed to investigate the influence of dehydration and plasma volume contraction on ECFVS markers and thyroid hormone serum concentrations, and to test the following two hypotheses: total T_3 (TT_3) and T_4 (TT_4) levels in dehydrated patients increase in proportion to the degree of fluid losses and the increases in T_3 and T_4 levels parallel those of ECFVS markers, and these alterations are rapidly reversible with rehydration.

Patient characteristics

The authors recruited 22 consecutive patients from October 1, 2004 to September 30, 2005 with no personal or family history of thyroid disease, goiter, or autoimmune diseases, who had not received irradiation to the head and neck or recent iodine-containing contrast agent exposure. Otherwise, patients did not present with renal or hepatic diseases and were not receiving any medication known to interfere with thyroid function or the measurement of thyroid hormone concentrations (amiodarone, dopamine, glucocorticoids, lithium, intravenous heparin, antiepileptic drugs, interferon-α, or interleukin-2). Patients were admitted to Centro Medico Teknon (Barcelona, Spain) with mild/moderate dehydration secondary to upper (3/22) or lower (4/22) gastrointestinal losses, in addition to miscellaneous/poor oral intake (15/22). The study included 16 women and 6 men, aged 66.3 ± 3.9 years (range, 48–88 years).

Methods

The following laboratory parameters were measured on admission, 48 to 72 hours after intravenous fluid therapy, and 3 months after hospital discharge: TT_4 (μg/dL), thyrotropin (mU/L), TT_3 (ng/dL), measured free T4 (FT_4; ng/dL), T_3-resin uptake (T_3RU), calculated FT_4 index (FT_4I; $T_4 \times T_3RU$), calculated free T_3 index (FT_3I; $T_3 \times T_3RU$), complete blood cell (CBC) count, and CHEM 23. CBC and CHEM 23 values were determined using commercial laboratory kits.

Serum T_4, T_3, and the thyroid hormone–binding index were measured with the use of kits from Abbott Laboratories (Abbott Park, Illinois). The serum-free T_4 index was calculated as the product of the serum T_4 concentration and the thyroid hormone–binding index value. Serum-free T_4 was measured by a two-step radioimmunoassay with the use of kits from Dia-Sorin (Stillwater, Minnesota). Serum thyrotropin was measured by fluoroimmunoassay with the use of kits from Wallac Oy (Turku, Finland). The lower limit of detectability with the assay was 0.002 μU/mL, and the normal range was 0.5 to 5.0 µU/mL. T_3RU was measured according to Sterling and colleagues [10]. The intra-assay coefficients of variation ranged from 1.2% to 3.5%.

The following alterations (change, relative change) in these parameters were calculated to determine the effects of hydration on thyroid hormone levels: change or Δ = concentration before − concentration after rehydration, and relative change = Δ/concentration before.

Statistical methods

Student's paired t test and Pearson's correlation were used. Values of $P<0.05$ were considered statistically significant. All calculations were performed using the SPSS 12.0 statistical package (SPSS Inc., Chicago, IL).

Results

Table 1 depicts the concentrations of ECFVS markers (serum urea nitrogen, creatine, uric acid, albumin, and hematocrit) and thyroid hormones at baseline (upon arrival at the emergency room [before]) and 48 to 72 hours thereafter (after), as well as the relative change. There were significant decreases in all ECFVS markers as well as in TT_4 and TT_3 and their free indexes (FT_4I and FT_3I). Thyrotropin values displayed a decrease that did not reach statistical significance. On the contrary, T_3RU concentrations exhibited a significant increase. Three months after discharge, ECFVS markers and thyroid hormone levels were nearly identical to those obtained after rehydration (data not shown).

Table 2 shows the degree of correlation (r) between the relative change of the 12 analyzed variables (BUN, creatine, uric acid, albumin, hematocrit,

Table 1
Extracellular fluid volume status markers and thyroid hormones

	Before	After	Relative change (%)	P
Bound urea nitrogen (mg/dL)	34.73 ± 4.02	16.00 ± 1.32	−54.00	1.70E-06
Creatinine (mg/dL)	1.82 ± 0.17	1.08 ± 0.08	−40.60	.00002
Uric acid (mg/dL)	7.22 ± 0.72	4.76 ± 0.41	−34.00	.000005
Albumin (g/dL)	3.73 ± 0.17	2.95 ± 0.12	−20.90	3.15E-05
Hematocrit (%)	40.50 ± 1.64	34.14 ± 1.45	−15.70	.00011
Total T_4 (µg/dL)	8.61 ± 0.50	6.93 ± 0.39	−19.50	6.03E-05
FT_4I	9.60 ± 0.74	8.43 ± 0.45	−12.18	.0339
Free T_4 (ng/dL)	1.56 ± 0.09	1.39 ± 0.08	−10.90	.00401
Total T_3 (ng/dL)	107.50 ± 7.95	88.05 ± 8.78	−18.09	.002961
FT_3I	119.04 ± 8.80	103.93 ± 8.23	−12.70	.0384
T_3RU	1.13 ± 0.06	1.25 ± 0.07	+10.62	.009806
Thyrotropin (mU/L)	1.67 ± 0.06	1.43 ± 0.24	−14.37	.050465

Table 2
Correlation matrix showing the Spearman's correlation (r) between the relative change of the 12 analyzed variables

	BUN	CREAT	URIC	ALB	HCT	T_4	FT_4I	FT_4	T_3	FT_3I	T_3RU	THYRO
ALB		0.5787*	0.4090*		0.3314	-0.0260	-0.5022*	-0.2079	0.4337	0.0362	0.8105**	0.3927*
T_3RU	-0.4688*	-0.5610*	-0.4518*	-0.8105**	-0.4832*	0.1457	0.7895**	0.1081	-0.3196	0.3645		0.1133
TT_4	0.5792*	0.2063	0.3351	-0.0026	0.4806*		0.7423**	0.040	0.4792*	0.4360*	0.1457	0.2127
TT_3	0.2366	0.1080	0.2443	0.4337	0.5805*	0.4792*	-0.0488	-0.3619		0.8759**	-0.3196	0.2198

Abbreviations: ALB, albumin; BUN, bound urea nitrogen; CREAT, creatinine; HCT, hematocrit; THYRO, thyrotropin; URIC, uric acid.

* $P < .01$.
** $P < .001$.

TT_4, FT_4I, FT_4, T_3, FT_3I, T_3RU, and thyrotropin) versus albumin, T_3RU, T_4, and T_3.

The relative change in albumin displayed a significant correlation with those observed in creatine, uric acid, FT_4I, TT_3, T_3RU, and thyrotropin. No correlations were found between the relative change in albumin and the changes observed in BUN, hematocrit, TT_4, FT_4, and FT_3I. The relative change in T_3RU correlated significantly with those of BUN, creatine, uric acid, albumin, hematocrit, and FT_4I. The relative change in TT_4 correlated significantly with those of BUN, hematocrit, uric acid, FT_4I, T_3, and FT_3I. The relative change in TT_3 correlated significantly with those of albumin, hematocrit, uric acid, TT_4, and FT_3I.

Discussion

The focus of this article is thyroid function assessment in the setting of dehydrated elderly outpatients. Dehydrated elderly patients are encountered commonly in emergency wards and outpatient clinics worldwide, given the increasing life expectancy of the population and the natural trend of the elderly to undergo dehydration. Moreover, a thyroid pathology is sought commonly in this age group when hyperadrenergic signs and symptoms dominate the clinical picture [11–13]. Some of the latter may be attributable to dehydration itself, which, in this particular setting, leads to plasma volume contraction (hypovolemia) and ensuing hemoconcentration. Thus, ECFVS markers show an increase in their plasmatic concentrations; this is also true for thyroid hormone concentrations because more than 99% of thyroid hormones are protein bound (TBG, albumin, transthyretin).

On admission, the entire panel of ECFVS markers (see Table 1) reflected mild to moderate dehydration. This condition was easily reversible and was corrected in 48 to 72 hours. Altogether, the degree of correlation between some (albumin, creatinine, uric acid) volume markers (see Table 2) displays an acceptable degree of internal consistency and serves as a proof of internal positive control.

Thyroid function tests must be interpreted with caution in a geriatric population, particularly with relation to the severity of the clinical state, and reference values should be determined for TT_3 and FT_4 in the ageing process [11,12]. Additionally, thyroid function tests can be altered by diabetes mellitus and obesity [14].

The extracellular fluid abnormalities of hypothalamic hypodipsia-hypernatremia syndrome are similar to those encountered in the authors' population, and were reported to be associated with similar alterations in thyroid function tests [15].

The classic thyroid abnormalities that are characteristic of the euthyroid sick syndrome (low T_3, low T_4, low thyrotropin, or all three) [16–30] were not present in any of the authors' patients. On the contrary, these values were in the normal-to-high range and decreased significantly by 19.5%, 18% and 14%, respectively, after 48 to 72 hours of intravenous fluid therapy. Additionally, the relative changes in TT_4 and TT_3 showed a significant positive correlation ($r = 0.4792$; $P < .01$; data not shown), which argues against the diagnosis of euthyroid sick syndrome, in which T_3 changes are predominant features, secondary to impaired peripheral ($D'5$) deiodinating enzymatic activity.

Moreover, the baseline T_3RU concentrations, their rapid increase ($+10.6\%$) after hydration (see Table 1), and the correlation with albumin changes (see Table 2) argues against the latter diagnosis [30].

The patient population in this study excluded patients who proceeded to the ICU (to exclude those who presented with serious, life-threatening non-thyroidal illnesses that could account for euthyroid sick syndrome) and those who presented with acute psychiatric illnesses to be taken into account for the interpretation of the thyroid as well as other hormonal levels [25,26,29]. Additionally, none of them was a known diabetic or obese.

The lack of correlation of relative changes in T_4 concentration with those of albumin can be explained by recalling basic physiology concepts; less than 15% of circulating TT_4 is bound to albumin [6–8], whereas most circulating T_4 is bound to globulins (mainly TBG). Because the dissociation constant of T_3 to albumin is markedly greater than that of T_4, it may account for the positive correlation between total and relative changes of T_3 and albumin levels (see Table 2).

The lack of correlation between the decrease in thyrotropin levels and the ECFVS markers and other thyroid hormone levels can be understood based on its brief plasma half-life (minutes). The data sampling was not accurate enough to detect subtle changes in the thyrotropin kinetics secondary to hemoconcentration and plasma volume contraction.

Ideally, thyroid hormone concentrations should have been measured before hospitalization to interpret the observed changes properly; nevertheless, it is likely that the observed changes in thyroid hormone concentrations were only transitory, because complete re-equilibrium between extracellular fluid volume and plasma volume was not completely achieved 48 to 72 hours after intravenous fluid therapy. Furthermore, thyroid hormone values 3 months later were nearly identical to those achieved at hospital discharge. Additionally, it must be taken into account that none of the thyroid values observed upon admission could have prompted the suspicion of subclinical hyperthyroidism. This drawback limits the usefulness of this finding in the clinical setting.

The authors have identified a unique, and, to the best of their knowledge, previously unreported reversible and factitious alteration in thyroid hormone concentration and function tests in patients who have contracted extracellular fluid volume. The latter, by itself, constitutes a new biochemical entity, different from that of euthyroid sick syndrome [25,26,29]; it should be considered when evaluating thyroid function in elderly patients who have volume contraction.

References

[1] Lowe GD. Blood rheology in general medicine and surgery. Baillieres Clin Haematol 1987; 1(3):827–61.

[2] Malarkey WB, Hall JC, Rice RR Jr, et al. The influence of age on endocrine responses to ultraendurance stress. J Gerontol 1993;48(4):134–9.

[3] Farber HW, Schaefer EJ, Franey R, et al. The endurance triathlon: metabolic changes after each event and during recovery. Med Sci Sports Exerc 1991;23(8):959–65.

[4] Van Stuijvenberg ME, Schabort I, Labadarios D, et al. The nutritional status and treatment of patients with hyperemesis gravidarum. Am J Obstet Gynecol 1995;172(5):1585–91.

[5] Lucke JN, Hall GN. Further studies on the metabolic effect of long distance riding: Golden Horseshoe Ride 1979. Equine Vet J 1980;12(4):189–92.

[6] Larsen PR. The thyroid. In: Wyngaarde JB, Smith LH, editors. Cecil textbook of medicine. 18th edition. Philadelphia: WB Saunders Co.; 1988. p. 1315–40.

[7] Pardridge WM. Transport of protein-bound hormones into tissues in vivo. Endocr Rev 1981;2(1):103–23.

[8] Utiger RD. The thyroid: physiology, hyperthyroidism, hypothyroidism, and the painful thyroid. In: Felig P, Baxter ID, Broadus AE, et al, editors. Endocrinology and metabolism. 2nd edition. New York: McGraw-Hill Book Co.; 1987. p. 389–472.

[9] Keane PM, Walker WHC, Thornton G, et al. Studies of thyroxine binding to plasma proteins in health and diseases. Clin Biochem 1986;19:52–7.

[10] Brent GA, Hershman JM. Thyroxine therapy in patients with severe non-thyroidal illness and low serum thyroxine concentration. J Clin Endocrinol Metab 1986;63:1–8.

[11] Blum CJ, Lafont C, Ducasse M, et al. Thyroid function tests in ageing and their relation to associated nonthyroidal disease. J Endocrinol Invest 1989;12(5):307–12.

[12] Simmon RJ, Simon JM, Demers LM, et al. Thyroid function in elderly hospitalized patients: effect of age and severity of illnesses. Arch Intern Med 1990;150:1249–53.

[13] Chopra IJ, Hershman JM, Pardridge WM, et al. Thyroid function in non-thyroidal illness. Ann Intern Med 1983;98:946–57.

[14] Proces S, Delgrange E, Vander Borght TV, et al. Minor alterations in thyroid-function tests associated with diabetes mellitus and obesity in outpatients without known thyroid illness. Acta Clin Belg 2001;56(2):86–90.

[15] Yamamoto T, Shimizu M, Fukuyama J, et al. Pathogenesis of extracellular fluid abnormalities of hypothalamic hypodipsia-hypernatremia syndrome. Endocrinol Jpn 1988;35(6): 915–24.

[16] Kaplan MM, Larsen PR, Crantz FR, et al. Prevalence of abnormal thyroid function tests in patients with acute medical illnesses. Am J Med 1982;72:9–16.

[17] Morley JE, Slag MF, Elson MK, et al. The interpretation of thyroid function tests in hospitalized patients. JAMA 1983;249:2377–9.

[18] Bayer MF. Free-thyroxine results are affected by albumin concentration and non-thyroidal illness. Clin Chim Acta 1983;130:391–6.

[19] Chopra IJ, Van Herle AJ, Teco GNC, et al. Serum free thyroxine in thyroidal and nonthyroidal illnesses: a comparison of measurements by radioimmunoassay, equilibrium dialysis, and free thyroxine index. J Clin Endocrinol Metab 1980;51:135–43.

[20] Csako G, Benson C, Ruddel M. On the albumin dependence of measurements of free thyroxine. I. Technical performance of seven methods. Clin Chem 1986;32:108–15.

[21] Csako G, Zweig MH, Glickman J, et al. Direct and indirect techniques for free thyroxine compared in patients withy nonthyroidal illness. II. Effect of prealbumin, albumin, and thyroxine-binding globulin. Clin Chem 1989;35:1655–62.

[22] Csako G, Zweig MH, Ruddel M, et al. Direct and indirect techniques for free thyroxine compared in patients with non-thyroidal illness. III. Analysis of interference variables by stepwise regression. Clin Chem 1990;36:645–50.

[23] Csako G, Zweig MH, Glickman J, et al. Direct and indirect techniques for free thyroxine compared in patients with non-thyroidal illness. I. Effect of free fatty acids. Clin Chem 1989;35:102–9.

[24] Konno N, Bamforth FJ. Concentrations of free thyroxine in serum during nonthyroidal illness-calculations or measurement? Clin Chem 1989;35:159–63.

[25] Melmed S, Geola FL, Reed AW, et al. A comparison of methods for assessing thyroid function in nonthyroidal illness. J Clin Endocrinol Metab 1982;54:300–6.

[26] Stockright JR. Guidelines for diagnosis and monitoring of thyroid disease: nonthyroidal illness. Clin Chem 1996;42:188–92.

[27] Slag MF, Morley JE, Elson MK, et al. Free thyroxine levels in critically ill patients. JAMA 1981;246:2702–6.

[28] Vermaak WJH, Kalk W, Zakolski WJ. Frequency of euthyroid sick syndrome as assessed by free thyroxine index and a direct free thyroxine assay. Lancet 1983;1:1373–5.

[29] Hay ID, Bayer MF, Kaplan MM, et al, for the Committee on Nomenclature of the American Thyroid Association. American Thyroid Association assessment of current free thyroid hormone and thyrotropin measurements and guidelines for future clinical assays. Clin Chem 1991;37:2002–8.

[30] Wehman RE, Gregerman RI, Burns WH, et al. Suppression of thyrotropin in the low-thyroxine state of severe nonthyroidal illness. N Engl J Med 1985;312:546–52.

ELSEVIER
SAUNDERS

Nurs Clin N Am 42 (2007) 135–138

NURSING
CLINICS
OF NORTH AMERICA

Index

Note: Page numbers of article titles are in **boldface** type.

Moving?

Make sure your subscription moves with you!

To notify us of your new address, find your **Clinics Account Number** (located on your mailing label above your name), and contact customer service at:

E-mail: elspcs@elsevier.com

800-654-2452 (subscribers in the U.S. & Canada)
407-345-4000 (subscribers outside of the U.S. & Canada)

Fax number: 407-363-9661

Elsevier Periodicals Customer Service
6277 Sea Harbor Drive
Orlando, FL 32887-4800

*To ensure uninterrupted delivery of your subscription, please notify us at least 4 weeks in advance of move.